ALLERGY ENVIRONMENT GUIDEBOOK

✦

New Hope and Help for Living and Working Allergy-Free

✦

JUDY L. BACHMAN, PH.D.

A Perigee Book

Perigee Books
are published by
The Putnam Publishing Group
200 Madison Avenue
New York, NY 10016

Library of Congress Cataloging-in-Publication Data

Bachman, Judy Lee.
   Allergy environment guidebook / Judy Lee Bachman.
      p. cm.
   Reprint. Originally published: Del Mar, Calif. : Health Services
Consultants, c1989.
   Includes bibliographical references.
   ISBN 0-399-51628-X
   1. Allergy—Popular works.   I. Title.
[RC584.B33   1990]   90-7314 CIP
616.97—dc20

ACKNOWLEDGMENTS
Karen Jacobs, Graphics
Elizabeth Burdette, Editing and Proofing
Donna Miceli, Editing
Laura Lehman, Typesetting, Layout

Printed in the United States of America

1 2 3 4 5 6 7 8 9 10

This book is printed on acid-free paper.
∞

TABLE OF CONTENTS

✦ PREFACE

The National Institutes of Health estimate that approximately 35 million Americans suffer from allergies — nine million of them from asthma. Annually, 35 million days are spent in bed as a result of asthma. Three million days of restricted activity, 6 million days of bed rest, and 3 million days of work lost all result from hay fever. Considering that one out of six people has allergy, a great impact on quality of life exists for a large number of people. Although medical science can usually pinpoint the causes of allergy in the individual sufferer, and a variety of medications are available to alleviate the symptoms, there is as yet no cure. Avoidance of the allergens is still the most important factor in preventing or controlling allergy symptoms, and this can involve major changes in person's environment and lifestyle.

Often the task seems overwhelming. The allergic person may feel "set apart" from society and denied the right to pursue a normal lifestyle to protect his or her health. After being told to eliminate dust from the home environment, allergy sufferers may envision a house bare of charm and comfort — one that resembles a sterile clinic more than a home. After being told to avoid pollen, molds, animal dander, and certain foods, they may picture a future without such simple pleasures as walks in the park, picnics, and family vacations. Such a future may seem bleak indeed, and it is not surprising that many people with newly diagnosed allergies experience some psychological difficulties in learning to cope with them.

It is possible, however, for allergic people to control their symptoms and still maintain comfortable homes and enjoyable lifestyles. Their homes will appear normal; only their closest friends will know that the surroundings are carefully selected to avoid allergens. The secret is in learning to create and maintain a balance between the environment and other factors that affect a person's health, primarily physical conditions and the way in which emotions are handled. This book is intended to serve as a guide to achieving such a balance. We can think of this as a state of total positive health.

1

✦

ALLERGY AND ITS IMPACT ON LIFESTYLE

WHAT IS ALLERGY?

If stepping outside on a beautiful spring day causes your nose to run and your eyes to itch and water, if the mere presence of a cat sends you into sneezing fits, or if biting into a ripe tomato causes you to break out in hives, you are probably a victim of allergies. In other words, your body produces an adverse reaction to substances in the environment that are normally considered harmless. When an allergic person is exposed to such a substance, known as an allergen or antigen, proteins called antibodies form in the blood and cause a chain of events that leads to the symptoms of allergy. When these antibodies react with the offending allergen, chemicals are released into the blood that affect organs or tissues in any part of the body.

IgE, one of the several different types of antibodies in the blood, plays a significant role in allergy. Allergy sufferers have a higher level of IgE than persons without allergies. This tendency for the body to make extra IgE is inherited. The IgE antibody attaches itself to specialized cells, called mast cells, that line the respiratory and intestinal tracts and tiny veins. Under normal circumstances, these cells protect the body against any foreign particles that may enter it. When IgE reacts with an allergen, mast cells release chemicals in an effort to destroy the foreign substance.

One of these chemicals is histamine. Large amounts of histamine are usually contained in the lining of the respiratory tract. Release of histamine can result in a variety of symptoms. If histamine is released from cells in the nose, for example, the nose begins to swell, run, and itch, and the person may begin to sneeze. If the eyes are affected, they may begin to swell, weep and itch. Reactions such as these are called "local" reactions because the symptoms are confined to the organs exposed to the allergen. Systemic, or whole-body, reactions can take place when the blood begins to circulate the chemicals throughout the body. The allergic person may then experience generalized fatigue or swelling, digestive discomfort or even asthma. In allergy's severest form, anaphylactic shock, the person collapses and can die in a few minutes. Only some people experience allergy. Research has not been able to explain why.

EVERYONE HAS A UNIQUE REACTION PATTERN

The kind of reaction a person has to a given allergen is unique to that person. Because the "target" organ or symptom location varies with the individual, several allergic persons, all sharing sensitivity to a given allergen, can be exposed to the substance with different results. For example, inhaling pollen may cause the itchy, runny nose of hay fever in one person and an asthma attack in another. A third person may break out in hives as a result of the pollen coming into contact with the skin.

To further complicate matters, a person who is allergic can react to the same allergen with different symptoms at different times, or with no symptoms, depending on the body's balance at the time of the exposure. If a person is overtired, for instance, or has recently been exposed to other allergens, the body's tolerance level may be exceeded when it faces a new exposure, and the reaction may be severe. If, on the other hand, resistance is high, the same person may have little or no reaction to the same allergen.

In the field of allergy, the term specific is frequently used to identify a particular substance, such as cat dander, that causes the body to react and release chemicals. If we could look at the IgE in the mast cells under a microscope when cat dander came near, we would see the IgE attach itself to the dander, and we would

	Seasonal pollen or mold allergy **Hayfever** or **Allergic Rhinitis**	**Year-Round Allergy** or **Allergic Rhinitis**	**Infections** or **Infectious Rhinitis**	**Physical Reaction** or **Vasomotor Rhinitis**
Seasonal Incidence	Present	Absent	Absent or worse in winter	Absent or worse in winter
Itching of Nose, Eyes Throat	Usual	Usual	Rare	Unusual
Sore Throat	Unusual	Usual	Usual	Unusual
Family History	65% or more	65% or more	Rare	Occasional
Red Eyes	Common	Common	Occasional	Occasional
Sore Skin Around Nose	Rare	Occasional	Usual	Rare
Red Throat	Rare	Occasional	Common	Rare
Swollen Glands in Neck	Occasional	Occasional	Usual	Rare
Thick Nasal Discharge	Absent	Absent	Common	Clear Common
Headache or Face Pain	Occasional	Occasional	Common	Occasional

Chart comparing vasomotor and allergic rhinitis

see the chemicals being released in an attempt to get rid of this foreign substance. In an allergic person, this reaction is specific. Every time the cat dander comes into contact with the cells, a reaction occurs.

It is obvious, then, that the subject of allergy is a complicated one. Detecting what allergens are causing the symptoms and learning to avoid allergens is the first step toward control of allergies. Maintaining a balance in daily life between the environment, emotions, and the physical condition becomes the ongoing lifestyle. When such a balance is achieved, a general state of well-being or total positive health is the natural result.

THE MOST COMMON TYPES OF ALLERGY

The most common kinds of allergy affect either the respiratory system or the skin. Although other kinds of symptoms have occasionally been traced to allergy, most allergy sufferers will recognize their symptoms in one or more of the following descriptions of specific allergic conditions:

Hay Fever

Allergic rhinitis, commonly called hay fever, is usually characterized by frequent sneezing, a stuffy or runny nose, and swollen, watery eyes. Itching of the nose, palate, throat, face and ears is also common. Some sufferers of hay fever feel tired, irritable, or chilly. Still others get headaches. Symptoms may be present continuously or only upon awakening or while the person is exposed to the allergen. Frequently, people who suffer from allergic rhinitis find they are also susceptible to infections of the ear or throat.

Allergic rhinitis can result from sensitivity to seasonal pollens or mold spores and may appear only during the spring, summer, or fall. It can develop as a reaction to environmental substances that are present year-round. People who suffer year-round from allergic rhinitis usually have milder symptoms than those who have seasonal attacks.

Another form of rhinitis, vasomotor rhinitis, develops as a

response to certain stimuli such as odors, pollutants, emotions, chilliness, fatigue, or humidity that are usually not thought of as allergens. A person suffering from allergic rhinitis may have vasomotor rhinitis as well. A skin test is often necessary to determine the source of the symptoms. A person with allergic rhinitis will usually show a positive reaction when the allergens are tested on the skin, whereas a person with the vasomotor form will not react.

It is a good idea for anyone who suffers from frequent cold symptoms to investigate the possibility of allergy, because "colds" are often allergies in disguise. Especially suspect are "little colds" that last only a day or two. An ordinary viral cold lasts more than a week and usually begins with a sore throat and fever.

Bronchial Asthma

Bronchial asthma is the technical term used to refer to spasms in the bronchial walls coupled with the formation of mucous. If this condition is ignored and untreated, it can result in chronic disabling disease. Infections such as pneumonia are not uncommon occurrences in the lives of asthmatic people.

Although wheezing is the most widely known symptom associated with asthma, a wheeze is not audible until the airway is already 50 percent constricted from spasm. Persons with mild asthma may never develop audible wheezes. They may, however, tire easily, experience shortness of breath, especially when exercising, and may have discomfort or tightness in the chest. A dry cough at night may be the only sign of the spasm.

Not all asthma is caused by allergy. A physician will be able to determine the cause by taking a medical history, conducting a physical examination, and running a few laboratory tests. Asthma that is caused by allergy, however, is generally considered the easiest kind to control.

Atopic, or allergic, asthma is usually caused by allergens of the inhalant variety, though occasionally by foods. In addition to allergens, an asthmatic person is especially sensitive to elements

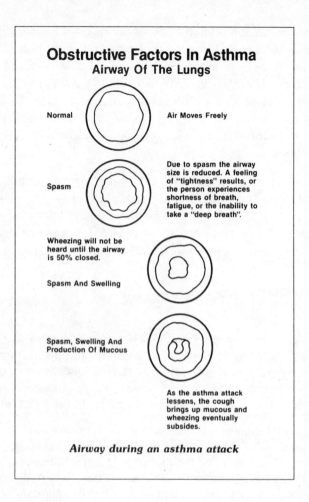

Obstructive Factors In Asthma
Airway Of The Lungs

Normal — Air Moves Freely

Spasm — Due to spasm the airway size is reduced. A feeling of "tightness" results, or the person experiences shortness of breath, fatigue, or the inability to take a "deep breath".

Wheezing will not be heard until the airway is 50% closed.

Spasm And Swelling

Spasm, Swelling And Production Of Mucous

As the asthma attack lessens, the cough brings up mucous and wheezing eventually subsides.

Airway during an asthma attack

in the environment that ordinarily do not affect other people. Such stimuli as cold air; changes in temperature, humidity, or barometric pressure; air pollution; exercise; odors or fumes; emotional stress; or even laughter, can affect an asthmatic adversely.

Prompt and proper medical treatment is critical to the well-being of a person who suffers from asthma, both to prevent future complications and to provide symptoms relief. With proper care, more than 90 percent of asthma sufferers can expect to attain relief from their symptoms. The remainder can anticipate significant improvement.

Eczema

Atopic dermatitis, commonly called eczema, is characterized by an inflammatory reaction of the skin caused by scratching and accompanied by severe itching. Three different forms of this allergic condition exist: infantile, juvenile, and adult. These are probably three phases of the same condition. Infantile eczema begins in infancy and usually clears up when the child is about two years old. Some youngsters have a flare-up of the condition at about the same time they go into puberty. Adult eczema usually appears before the person is 30 years old.

Because skin eruptions are difficult to diagnose, it is always advisable to consult a dermatologist when symptoms persist. Skin tests are difficult to perform on patients with eczema; the skin of such a patient is so sensitive it often overreacts. Frequently, food-elimination diets can help determine the source of the symptoms, especially in infants.

The actual cause of eczema is unclear. Studies have shown that more than 50 percent of children with eczema develop respiratory allergy before they are 10 years old.

Hives and Angioedema

Hives and angioedema are different forms of the same condition. Although both are characterized by swellings under the surface of the skin, hives affect the upper skin surfaces, whereas in angioedema the deeper tissues are involved. Thus, hives tend to itch because the swelling affects nerve endings near the skin's surface. In angioedema, no itching is felt.

Among the agents thought to cause an attack of hives or angioedema are drugs, foods, stress, such inhalant allergens as pollens or dust, infections, disease of the connective tissues, and insect bites or stings. Angioedema can occur as part of the shock reaction of people who are allergic to insect bites or stings. Because the internal swelling of angioedema can cause breathing passages to close, prompt medical attention is essential when such a reaction occurs.

Anaphylaxis

Anaphylaxis, an unusually strong reaction to an allergen, is life-threatening. Stories about people who have died from an insect sting are not unusual. People sensitive to insect stings may not have a reaction the first time they are stung because the antibodies that cause the reaction have not been previously developed before the sting occurs. However, often a second sting results in a severe reaction.

A normal reaction to stings includes pain, redness, swelling, itching, and a hot feeling at the site of the sting. After a few hours, all the symptoms disappear.

A person allergic to stinging insects may experience unusual swelling or hives, shortness of breath, wheezing, faintness, or, in its severest form, a drop in blood pressure and collapse.

Anaphylaxis can also occur in people who are allergic to drugs and medicines such as penicillin. A person who is suspect for such a reaction can be tested to confirm it. A physician can provide the appropriate prevention and treatment program.

WHO SUFFERS FROM ALLERGY?

According to the statistics compiled by the National Institute of Allergy and Infectious Disease, one in six people has allergy. This translates to 35.3 million people. Of those affected, 14.6 million have hay fever, 8.9 million have asthma, and 11.8 million have other forms of allergy such as eczema, hives, or swelling or reactions to food, medications, or insect bites.

Between 2,000 and 4,000 asthma deaths occur annually, a tragic loss considering that 98 percent of the asthmatics are now able to have their condition controlled by treatment and education.

The impact that asthma and allergy has on the quality of life is also dramatic. Each year, 35 million days are spent in bed as a result of asthma, and 28 million days of restricted activity, and 3 million lost work days are experienced by those who suffer from hay fever.

According to the National Center for Health Statistics, the expense of asthma and allergies in 1975 was $170 million for hospital care, $224 million for physician services, and $196 million for medications. Hay fever sufferers spent $224 million on physician services and $297 million on drugs. The cost of medical care since 1975 has risen sharply; therefore, the current numbers would be multiples of the 1975 numbers.

Children tend to have asthma more than adults. Surveys indicate that education, occupation, or income does not influence the prevalence of asthma.

The allergic family is a common occurrence. If one parent is allergic, a child has a one in four chance of developing allergy; if both parents are allergic the probability increases to two out of three.

Occupational allergic diseases are coming to the forefront of our awareness. Recently, it has been discovered that workplace ailments are more prevalent than previously thought. It is not clear if some of them are unique sensitivities or if some of them are allergic responses. Nevertheless, the workplace environment will become more and more an issue.

The total cost of these incurable immunologic diseases has been estimated by the Asthma and Allergy Foundation to be $4 billion in 1981. The cost of medical services was estimated to be $2 billion a year.

The costs related to lost wages probably exceed $8 million a year just for hay fever and asthma. Allergy plays a major part in our society.

2
THE NATURE OF ALLERGY

A great many persons have no idea of the relationship between the cause and the symptoms of their allergy. This may be due partly to a lack of awareness; however, the biggest part is due to the nature of allergy.

It is not uncommon for the signs and symptoms of allergy to change from time to time as a person progresses through different stages of life. Symptoms can even disappear for a year or two, perhaps permanently. A person is not necessarily permanently allergic but probably always retains the capacity for allergy.

The explanation for these changes or the disappearance of allergy symptoms varies in each individual. A reduction of symptoms or remission may be related to a person's physical condition, emotional state, or environment.

For example, if a person is receiving allergy shots, the body is building its own resistance to the allergens the person is exposed to. Or a physician may have prescribed medications that prevent symptoms by blocking or balancing certain chemicals in the body. Other aspects related to the body's physical condition such as dietary intake or a physical fitness program can also influence the degree of symptoms.

Age can play a part. All the time we hear about children who "outgrow" their allergies. Nobody knows for sure, but growth may result in a better physical balance that brings about the end of symptoms. The capacity for developing allergy is always there. For some, puberty may be the beginning of symptoms — or the childbearing years or middle or late life. A person may be miserable for a couple of weeks out of his or her entire lifetime and never experience symptoms of allergy again.

When it comes to environment, if a person who has an allergy to ragweed moves to an area where ragweed does not grow, the person may be symptom-free. There are case histories of children in military families who moved every two years and never experienced allergy. However, at the age of 10, when their families had stayed at one location for four years, the children developed allergies to the specific pollens found at that location. Because it takes approximately two years to acquire allergies to allergens in a new geographical location, the children escaped symptoms for many years.

Some people who have the potential for symptoms of allergy may not have problems until they experience a stressful period in their lives. It is possible that the stress affects the immune system and results in the appearance of allergy symptoms. Emotional experiences, happy or sad, can trigger the balance that seems to protect a person from suffering symptoms.

Colds frequently are blamed for allergy. Colds start out with a sore throat and fever and usually last 10 days. Anything that is a variation of this is suspect for allergy. A person who gets a "cold" every August or who gets a cold that lasts a few days or a whole month is probably an allergic person.

Sometimes it is easy to detect a food allergy because symptoms may be prominent within seconds after the food is eaten. The mouth may itch or begin to swell. Other reactions to food may result in tiredness, low energy, and headache for a day or two after the suspect food is eaten. These allergies are difficult to identify.

DO YOU HAVE AN ALLERGY?

If you suspect you have an allergy but have not recognized what causes symptoms, the following assessment will provide a guideline for allergy sources. Fill in the blanks or check the columns.

SELF-ASSESSMENT FOR ALLERGY AWARENESS

FAMILY HISTORY:

Family history is positive for allergy in 65 percent of cases. The types of allergy are as follows:

1• **Asthma** is characterized by chronic cough, episodes of loud breathing, history of pneumonia or bronchitis, chest colds or cough after exercise.

2• **Hay fever** may result in watering or itching of the eyes or nose. These symptoms may occur year-round or during a specific season or time. For example, sneezing several times in a row in the morning or during an exposure to an allergen such as a cat is common.

3• **Eczema** is characterized by itching of the skin. In children, the itching is usually behind the knees or behind the elbows, wrists, or ankles. The neck or cheeks are usually red. The skin becomes irritated and red from scratching and can eventually weep fluid.

FAMILY MEMBER   **TYPE OF ALLERGY**

_____ Mother   _____

_____ Father   _____

_____ Sisters/Brothers   _____

                                     _____

_____ Your children or   _____
        children of your siblings
                                     _____

CAUSES:

ANIMALS

☐ Cats   ☐ Birds   ☐ Guinea Pigs   ☐ Hamsters

☐ Dogs   ☐ Horses   ☐ Other (Name) _____

SPECIFIC ROOMS IN YOUR HOME

Experiencing symptoms in certain rooms in the home may indicate allergy to dust, molds, fibers or materials found there.

☐ Living room   ☐ Bathroom   ☐ Bedroom

☐ Attic   ☐ Basement   ☐ Garage

☐ Other Rooms (Name)

_____ _____ _____

_____ _____ _____

FOODS

List foods that cause symptoms such as burning in the mouth, digestive upset, colic, headache, tightness in the chest, or swelling around the lips, mouth, or throat:

_____ _____ _____

_____ _____ _____

SEASONS

Experiencing symptoms during any of the following seasons may indicate allergy to the items listed.

_____   Spring (grasses, tree pollens)

_____   Summer (grasses, weeds)

_____   Fall (weeds, molds)

_____   Winter (molds, tree pollen in mild climates)

Allergy symptoms at specific locations or situations

_____ Windy days (pollen, molds)

_____ Warm days (pollutants, pollens, molds)

_____ Country (pollens, molds)

_____ Farms (animals, pollens, molds)

_____ Circus (animals, molds, environmentals)

_____ Zoo (animals, molds)

_____ Mountains (pollens)

_____ Beach (molds)

_____ Outside home (pollens, molds)

_____ Inside home (environmentals, molds)

_____ Motels, hotels (molds, animals, environmentals)

_____ Old buildings (environmentals, molds)

_____ School
(animals, art supplies, chemicals, environmentals)

_____ Work (environmentals, pollutants,
chemicals used in the workplace, etc.)

_____ Rooms where people smoke

Certain activities

_____ Camping (pollens, molds;
environmentals in tent structure)

_____ Gyms, auditoriums (environmentals, molds)

_____ Boats (environmentals, molds)

_____ Outdoor sports (pollens, molds)

Medicine or Drugs

_____ Over-the-counter medications

BRAND	COLOR	TABLET OR SPANSULE	LIQUID-FLAVOR
_____	_____	_____	_____
_____	_____	_____	_____
_____	_____	_____	_____

_____ Marijuana (either smoking or being around it)

_____ Street drugs

_____ Daily medications (fillers, dyes, and capsule contents)

List brand, color of tablets (include vitamins):

BRAND	COLOR	TABLET OR SPANSULE	LIQUID-FLAVOR
_____	_____	_____	_____
_____	_____	_____	_____
_____	_____	_____	_____
_____	_____	_____	_____
_____	_____	_____	_____

BEYOND AWARENESS—
SELECTING YOUR OPTIONS

Now that you have completed the assessment, you may be more aware of the sources of your allergies. If you could not answer some of the questions, the assessment will serve as a guideline to what to watch for in the future.

The term allergy evokes different responses in different persons. For years there has been an attitude that allergy symptoms are a "state of mind." It is true that persons can influence their bodily functions, but most have not developed such skills. Chapter One covered the actual physical causes for allergy that people who make these statements do not know. Unfortunately this attitude has had detrimental effects, especially on growing children.

A child who constantly has a stuffy nose is forced to breath through the mouth, resulting in an open-mouth, gaping appearance. The facial structure actually changes over time. An overbite can result from a constant diversion of normal blood flow in the face. Bags under the eyes give any allergic person a tired

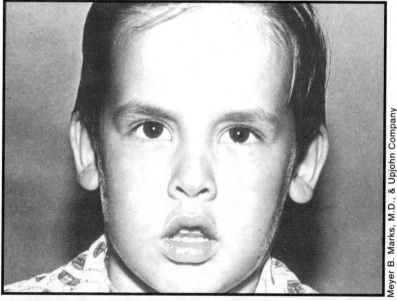

Meyer B. Marks, M.D., & Upjohn Company

Mouth breathing (*allergic gaping*). This child, aged 4 years, has had perennial allergic rhinitis since early infancy and has been a mouth breather since birth.

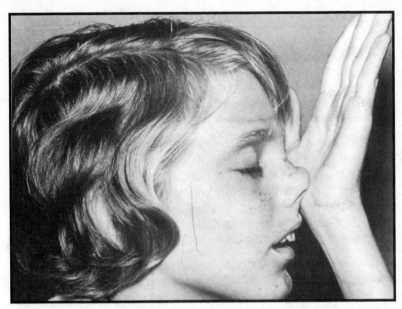

Allergic salute. The patient pushes the nose upward and backward to relieve itching and free edematous turbinates from contact with the septum, thus allowing freer passage of air. Child, aged 11 years, with perennial allergic rhinitis since age 2.

unattractive appearance. These facial appearances frequently bring comments that the child is dumb!

Chest deformities can develop in children who have untreated asthma. Over a period of time, air trapped in the lungs tends to push the rib cage outward. In addition, untreated asthma may result in repeated infections or permanent damage to the lung tissue, which could later result in emphysema.

Of even more importance is the psychological impact of untreated allergy on sufferers and those around them. Children who are constantly wiping their noses or coughing or who are grouchy because of not feeling well become an annoyance to others. Rejection occurs at school or at home. Some teachers either tend to isolate allergic children or go to the other extreme and expect an asthmatic child to be able to run the track every day. Sometimes the stress from a child's symptoms becomes such a focus in a family that normal family relations break down. As a result, resentment or frustration builds up against the child.

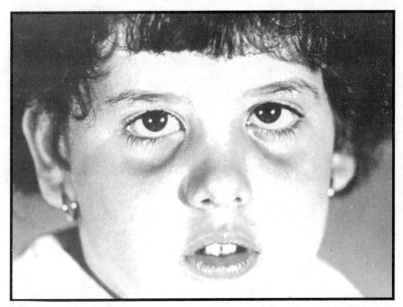

Allergic shiners in child, aged 4 years, with pronounced perennial allergic rhinitis due chiefly to foods and inhalants.

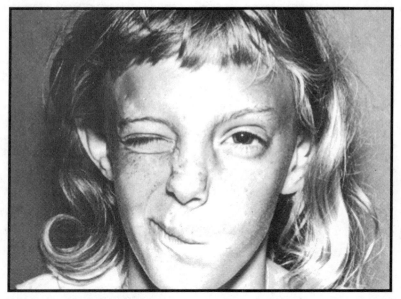

Mouth Wrinkling. Another facial grimace for the relief of nasal itching. Note puffy lower eyelids secondary to spasm of musculus tarsalis.

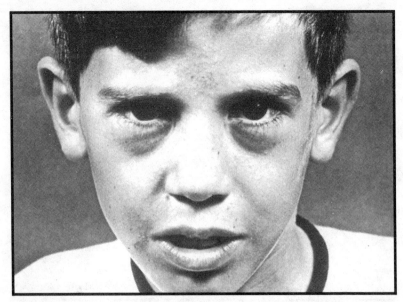

Allergic shiners in child, aged 8 years, with perennial allergic rhinitis and bronchial asthma since age 3. Note the "bags" (infraorbital edema) resulting from spasm of the unstriated muscle of Muller.

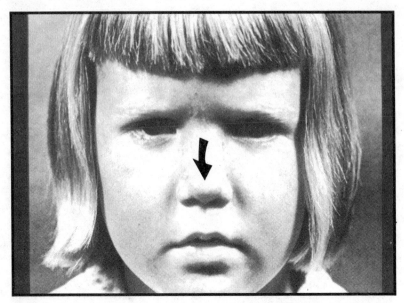

Transverse nasal crease in child, aged 6 years, with severe perennial allergic rhinitis since age 3 and recurrent attacks of pneumonia with bronchial asthma since age 4. (Arrow indicates crease.)

Such a family can benefit from child and family counseling to restore normal relations and to learn how to cope with the frustrations resulting from allergy.

The degree of your symptoms can be a guide to the options you will want to select. First of all, how severe are your symptoms?

If they are only an occasional mild annoyance and you are aware of what causes them, you have several choices: Avoid the known allergen, take over-the-counter antihistamines, ask your physician's advice, or ignore your symptoms.

If, however, your everyday living is affected, here are some indicators that might be worth checking. If you answer yes to any of these questions, you will probably benefit from an allergy workup.

☐ Do you use more than one box of tissues per week?

☐ Do you miss work or school because of your allergy?

☐ Do you miss sleep because your symptoms bother you at night?

☐ Are you not working at your capacity because you feel ill?

☐ Would you rather stay home than experience symptoms that occur when you participate in an activity such as mowing the lawn, or attending a smoky meeting?

SELECTING A PHYSICIAN

You have many options in selecting a physician to help you feel good again. First of all, you want to find one who will work with you, not just dictate your treatment program. Your family physician may refer you to an allergist. If you have a mild problem, your physician may recommend a medication or environmental changes before referring you to an allergist.

Many different kinds of physicians treat allergy. Some have very little training in the field and rely on skin tests to reveal what your allergies may be. Board-certified allergists receive a total of nine years of training: four years of medical school, three years in internal medicine or pediatrics. In addition, to receive certification, the physician must serve two years as a fellow in a program approved by the American Academy of Allergy and Immunology. These physicians must complete final tests conducted by the Academy. This expertise is recommended for anyone suffering significant allergy. If you are an asthmatic, you could be treated by a pulmonologist who has special training in allergy. Unfortunately, as in all fields of health, some testing and treatment methods are questionable. A number of methods for testing are not recognized by the American Academy of Allergy and Immunology. They are mentioned here to provide an understanding of why they are not accepted so that you can be better informed should you choose one of these methods.

CONTROVERSIAL TESTING METHODS

The American Academy of Allergy and Immunology reviewed the following allergy tests in response to a request by the National Center for Health Care Technology. In each case, the test was found to be ineffective and controversial and should be reserved for experimental uses. Be sure to question your physician if he or she recommends any of these tests.

Cytotoxicity Testing (Bryan's Test)

This blood test claims that the presence of a specific allergen will reduce the white blood count. It claims to diagnose food and inhalant allergies.
The American Academy of Allergy and Immunology cited a number of studies that led them to conclude that there is no proof this test is effective in diagnosing food and inhalant allergies. They further added that these tests should be labeled experimental.

Urine Autoinjection Therapy (Autogenous Urine Immunization)

Urine, collected and handled with special techniques, is injected back into the patient. Various reactions can occur, from redness at the site of the injection to severe physical reactions. This therapy is not considered standard medical practice, and it has not been proven effective by published studies. It is considered potentially dangerous for several reasons. The Academy could not identify any rationale or immunologic basis for this treatment.

Skin Titration (Rinkel Method)

In this procedure an injection of an allergen is placed beneath the skin in different strengths. The strength that causes the weakest skin reaction is then determined to be the starting dose. A therapeutic end dose, a given dose required to relieve allergy symptoms, is calculated from the weakest skin reaction.

The Academy's position is that this method does aid the physician as a rough guide for the beginning dose for immunotherapy. It is not a guide for determining the end dose for therapy. Controlled studies have shown that the end-point dilution does not demonstrate therapeutic effect. They also stated that this method should be reserved for experimental use.

Provocative and Neutralization Testing (Subcutaneous)

In this technique, an injection of the allergen is placed beneath the skin in a dose strong enough to elicit symptoms. Another injection of a weaker or stronger amount of the allergen is given immediately following to relieve or neutralize the provoked symptoms.

The Academy's position is that this method has no plausible rationale or immunologic basis. This method was tested and shown ineffective. This method should be used only in controlled experiments.

Provocative Testing (Sublingual)

Drops of allergens that are in a measured extract are placed under the tongue. After ten minutes, if the patient has symptoms, the physician administers a neutralizing dose. This is supposed to stop symptoms.

The Academy states that no studies are known to support this technique, and there are no immunologic reasons to explain "neutralizing effects." Until studies are conducted, this method is unproven and should be limited to research purposes only.

For more information on these tests, you can contact the American Academy of Allergy and Immunology.

THE ALLERGY WORKUP

The allergy workup consists of a very detailed history, tests, treatment plan, education, and follow-up. When taking the history, the physician will ask questions about cause-and-effect reactions that are similar to the material in the Self-Assessment presented earlier. Early childhood illnesses, family history, and lifestyle will all be covered. From this information the physician can interpret your history for medical significance. For an example, see the chart of a six-month history given by a mother and medically interpreted by the physician. Once this history is complete, a physical examination and some tests will complete your workup. Some tests are to establish the current level of certain physical functions. These tests, called baseline tests, can be used as a basis for comparison for any future tests. Such tests might include breathing tests to measure lung functions. Allergy skin tests will also be part of the workup.

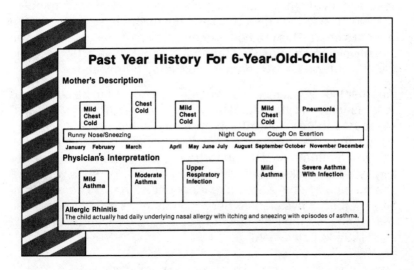

Graphic of history and interpretation

One type of skin test is called a scratch test. Allergens are suspended in a fluid that is dropped on the skin. A tiny scratch is made over the area to see if the skin reacts to the allergen.

It takes 10 to 30 minutes for a hive-like bump or a reddened area to appear. When such a reaction occurs, it is measured against a "control." The control, a drop of saline on the skin and a scratch, should not result in a bump or redness. If it does, it indicates that the skin is quite sensitive to being irritated. The second control, a drop of histamine and a scratch, should result in a wheal and redness. This indicates how and if the skin reacts. These controls influence decisions about which tests are positive and which ones are not.

Sometimes scratch skin tests do not result in a reaction. This may be due to the concentration of the allergen in the fluid, to the potency of the fluid, or to other causes that can influence these tests. If the person has a history of symptoms with reaction to specific allergens and the scratch test is negative or questionable, it is important to confirm this negative reaction by an intradermal skin test. In intradermal tests, a tiny amount of a measured concentration of the allergen is injected under the skin of the upper arm. The skin raises up slightly to form a bump when it reacts to an allergen. This reaction usually takes 5 to 15 minutes to develop. It is then measured and the reaction is entered on the patient's chart. This method is considered more reliable and gives the physician conclusive information about the starting dosage level in future allergy shots, should they be needed.

Another test frequently used but still considered to be somewhat less sensitive is the radioallergosorbent test (RAST). This test measures the amount of IgE antibody in the blood. It is more costly and time-consuming than other tests. It is useful, however, in certain situations. Persons who have severe skin diseases or highly reactive skin, very young children, and persons who have the potential to have severe reactions to skin tests benefit from this method. Physicians other than allergists tend to use these tests because their offices are not set up for skin testing, and the RAST is convenient.

ALLERGY SKIN TESTS RESULTS— WHAT DO THEY MEAN?

If you look at your allergy test sheet, you will see that allergens, especially pollens and molds, are frequently listed in Latin, with their common names following. Your physician will explain the results. Although you may find it difficult to remember what the Latin terms mean, they indicate the species of plants or animals used in the tests. Each species tested has two Latin names. The first one, capitalized, is the genus, and the second, uncapitalized, is the particular species. For instance, *Aspergillus fumigatus* is a fungus from the genus *Aspergillus*, which includes seven species; fumigatus is one of these seven. This system of biological classification is used for all plants and animals. The significance in understanding these classifications is that there are biological relationships within genuses and cross-reactions can occur. A cross-reaction can be described as a allergy reaction to one or more species of a genus. See "**Molds**" in Chapter Three.

An example of the family relationships is the legume family. Legumes include peanuts, beans, lentils, soybeans, and peas. According to your skin tests, you may be allergic to peanuts; however, an exposure to peas or beans has the potential to cause a reaction as well. This potential could include exposure to the pollen, the plant, or the food from this family. These botanical families are included in the index in the back of the book.

Suppose you see that you are allergic to *Ulmus Americana* or American elm. The next step is to learn about the elm and to determine how important it is in your environment. You may live in a grove of elm trees and find you cannot conveniently avoid them. Or you may find there are no elms in your neighborhood. In the first case, you may choose to get allergy shots if your physician recommends them, to take a vacation or stay inside an air-conditioned house during the pollen season, to move, or to take medications during the pollen season. If there are no elms around your home, you should determine how prevalent elms are in your area. It may be that most neighborhood streets are lined with them. In that case, your physician will probably recommend shots and medication. Although skin tests are generally considered reliable at pinpointing an allergy, they are not 100 percent foolproof.

Once all of these data are complete, the allergist will discuss treatment alternatives. In some cases, avoidance of the allergens is simple, and that is all that needs to be done. However, it is usually not that easy. Some symptoms may require medications.

In this day of taking medicine only when necessary, the allergic person may run into difficulty. In some allergy conditions, it is very important to follow the prescribed medication directions to prevent severe reactions. Frequently, allergy patients do not understand this and take medicine only when they feel bad.

Once your allergy symptoms are under control with medications, you can begin an avoidance program and learn more about balancing your symptoms. If you are going to start allergy shots, the medications can be reduced after a few months. As your allergy symptoms are reduced with the shots, your physician usually will be able to reduce your medications as you improve.

Allergy shots, medicine, and avoidance are usually the first choices to be made in balancing your lifestyle. After you are comfortable with these first choices, it is time to set goals for total positive health and lifestyle.

WHAT IS TOTAL POSITIVE HEALTH?

While modifying your environment to make it as allergen-free as possible, it is essential to your well-being to pay attention to your whole self, not just your allergies. It is important to recognize that environment is only one of the factors involved in keeping your life in balance. Important too are the state of your emotions and the general physical condition of your body.

In the past, the primary emphasis of medical science has been on curing disease. More and more, however, physicians are beginning to recognize how important it is for patients to participate in maintaining a state of positive health. Instead of viewing a patient as the host for a diseased heart, for instance, physicians who embrace the philosophy of positive health are now recognizing that the whole person — habits, personality, feelings, and stresses — plays a significant role in a person's ability to recover or prevent further illness. In other words, such a physician encourages patients to take responsiblity for their health by developing a positive lifestyle. The role of proper diet, appropriate exercise, and reduction of stress in the prevention of heart disease has been well-publicized. Less known is the fact that those same factors, combined with an appropriate modification of the

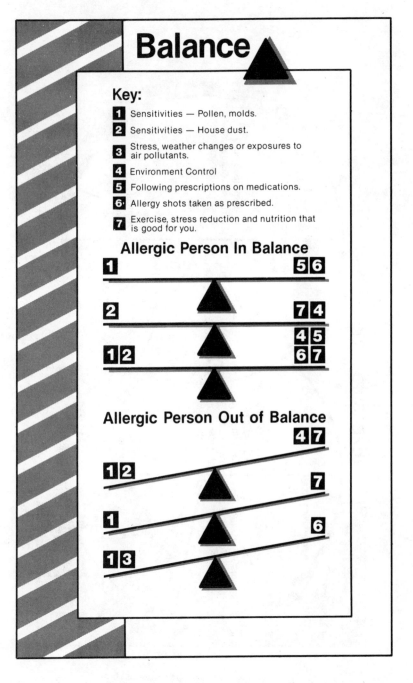

Balance

Key:

1 Sensitivities — Pollen, molds.

2 Sensitivities — House dust.

3 Stress, weather changes or exposures to air pollutants.

4 Environment Control

5 Following prescriptions on medications.

6 Allergy shots taken as prescribed.

7 Exercise, stress reduction and nutrition that is good for you.

Allergic Person In Balance

Allergic Person Out of Balance

Factors contributing to balance and inbalance in the life of an allergic person.

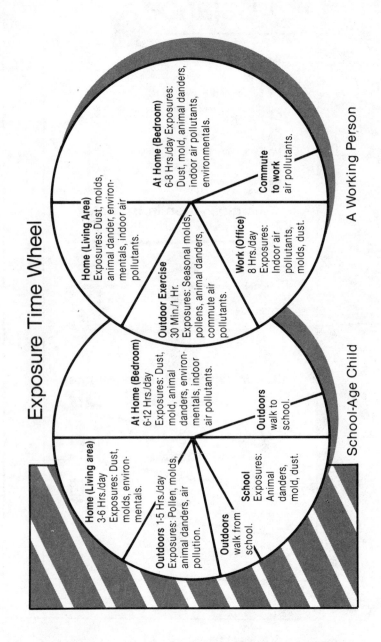

Exposure Time Wheel

A Working Person

Home (Living Area)
Exposures: Dust, molds, animal dander, environmentals, indoor air pollutants.

At Home (Bedroom)
6-8 Hrs./day Exposures: Dust, mold, animal danders, indoor air pollutants, environmentals.

Commute to work
air pollutants.

Work (Office)
8 Hrs./day Exposures: Indoor air pollutants, molds, dust.

Outdoor Exercise
30 Min./1 Hr. Exposures: Seasonal molds, pollens, animal danders, commute air pollutants.

School-Age Child

At Home (Bedroom)
6-12 Hrs./day Exposures: Dust, mold, animal danders, environmentals, indoor air pollutants.

Outdoors
walk to school.

Home (Living area)
3-6 Hrs./day Exposures: Dust, molds, environmentals.

Outdoors 1-5 Hrs./day Exposures: Pollen, molds, animal danders, air pollution.

Outdoors
walk from school.

School
Exposures: Animal danders, mold, dust.

Graph showing contrasting times of exposure to allergens for the school-age child and the working individual.

environment, play a significant part in the prevention or alleviation of symptoms of allergy.

For an allergic person, achieving and maintaining a balance in physical and emotional conditions can mean the difference between illness and health. Understanding and controlling the interplay between exposure to allergens and lifestyle can seem a bit overwhelming. However, like any other new concept, it becomes a relatively simple matter after the initial effort is made. The payoff in terms of feeling better can make it all seem worthwhile. There are several components involved in balancing your lifestyle. Daily living patterns may expose you to different allergens. Reviewing these lifestyle components and daily patterns is the first step toward bringing about a balance that results in total positive health.

This book focuses on just one of the components of positive health: the creation of an allergen-free environment. Lifestyle, stress, and health risk will be introduced; however, the other components, physical conditioning and nutrition, are well covered in books already on the shelves.

3
✦
THE ALLERGENS

Approximately 80 to 90 percent of allergies in adults are caused by inhalants such as pollens, molds, animal danders, and house dust. Twenty percent of allergies in children are caused by substances they eat or drink. In both adults and children less than 10 percent of allergies are caused by insect stings or contact allergy.

The environment plays an especially significant role in the well-being of an allergic person. Although most persons are affected by such natural forces as changes in temperature, humidity, and barometric pressure, all of which tax the body's ability to keep itself in balance, the allergic person faces additional environmental hazards. These are, of course, the allergens.

Briefly, these allergens consist of a large variety of gases, liquids, and solids. All of these can produce specific antibody responses that result in symptoms when an allergic person comes into contact with them. Not all allergic persons are sensitive to all of the allergens. However, exposure to some of these substances will result in the development of allergic symptoms for some people.

Allergens can be divided into five categories:

1 Inhalants.

Inhalants consist of dusts, particles, or vapors found in the air. These might include animal danders, feathers, vegetable seeds and fibers, pollens, molds, inhaled medications, and such odorous materials as perfumes.

2 Ingestants.

Ingestants include anything that may be eaten or drunk such as food, drinks, or medicines.

3 Injectants.

Injectants are anything that is injected into the body, such as medication or vaccines. Animal or insect bites or stings also introduce the allergen via the injection route.

4 Contactants.

Contactants include substances that touch or come in contact with the skin, such as clothing, plants, metals, woods, plastics, lotions, and leather.

5 Infectants.

Organisms that either infect the body or grow normally in it may result in symptoms of allergy. These include bacteria, fungi, and parasites such as worms or protozoa.

POLLENS

Pollens are found literally everywhere in the world. However, some places have more plants than others, depending on the terrain and climate. In the United States, many places produce great amounts of pollen that are carried by the wind. This is important; only wind-borne pollens affect allergy sufferers, causing hay fever. Tropical areas, such as Central America, have plants that depend upon pollination by insects. Because of the humidity in the tropics, these pollens are too heavy to be carried by the wind.

Wind pollens are very light. In fact, when studied under a microscope, they appear shaped for flight. The plants that produce these pollens grow in temperate regions and vary from place to place. However, for a plant to signficantly affect allergy sufferers, it must possess several characteristics. First, it must be seed bearing. This includes evergreens and flowering plants. This does *not* include flowers that have insect attractants such as nectar, odor, or color. Nor does it include ferns, mosses, or algae. Plants also must produce large amounts of pollen and inhabit a large area to cause problems for allergy sufferers. This does not mean, however, that the elm in the yard of an allergic person will not cause symptoms. One tree in a small area may be significant in that person's environment. Finally, as mentioned previously, the plant must produce pollen that's light enough to be carried by the air.

Any plant possessing most of these characteristics can cause hay fever. For a detailed listing of trees, grasses, and weeds that cause allergic symptoms in the United States and Canada, see the Appendix on page 187.

MOLDS

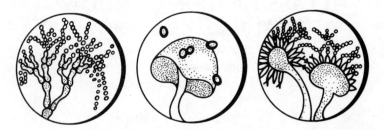

Fungi, or molds, are another area of major concern. Because molds are everywhere in nature, they are very difficult to remove from the environment. The term mold is generally accepted to include all small nonparasitic fungi. Fungi range in size from the single-celled microscopic yeasts to giant multicellular mushrooms and smut balls. Molds affect the allergic person in two ways. Some molds flourish at certain times of year, similar to pollen seasons, and thus cause the symptoms only at these times. Other molds are always present in the everyday living environment, for example, in buildings, boats, and food. These molds cause symptoms year-round.

The part of a mold that causes allergy is the reproductive part, the spore, which is produced in great abundance. Spores, the seeds of molds, are lightweight and easily wind-borne. With the right climate, temperature, and other conditions, mold spores can germinate by the thousands. Ideal conditions usually include warm weather and increased humidity. Most thrive in warm, dark, damp areas. They grow best at temperatures of 70 to 90 degrees Fahrenheit. Some are killed by higher temperatures. Many can survive a freezing winter.

Molds play a very important part in life cycles. Molds assist in the rotting of plants and trees. For example, after the molds rot dying plants and trees, the decayed remains help to build soil, making it possible to grow more plants. Molds can be both "good" and "bad." Some molds cause illness, and others, such as penicillin, cure illness. Molds are used to develop the flavor of wines and cheeses as well as spoil them. Just as pollens are categorized into biological groups, molds that cause allergy are divided into six families.

CLASSIFICATION OF MOLDS THAT CAUSE ALLERGY

CLASS	ORDER/FAMILY	GENUS
Phycomycetes	Zygomycetes	*Mucor*
		Rhizopus
Ascomycetes		*Saccharomyces*
		Chaetomium
Basidiomycetes		*Merulius*
		Ustilaginales
		Uredinales
Deuteromycetes	Sphaeropsidales	*Phoma*
	Moniliaceae	*Aspergillus*
		Penicillium
		Botrytis
		Monilia
		Mycogone
		Paecilomyces
		Trichoderma
		Gliocladium
	Dematiaceae	*Alternaria*
		Cladosporium
		(Hormodendrum)
		Helminthosporium
		Spondylocladium
		Stemphylium
		Nigrospora
		Pullularia
	Tuberculariacea	*Fusarium*
		Epicoccum
	Cryptococcaeae	*Rhodotorula*
		Cryptococcus

Seasonal Molds

The most commonly distributed seasonal molds are those that are part of the life cycles of crops and foliage. In the northern United States, plant debris begins to increase in late spring with the help of increased humidity and warmer weather. This gradual increase continues until the first frost of the fall.

In the southern United States, the so-called seasonal molds are found almost year-round. Molds can be present where winter crops are harvested, when soil is cultivated, and even in irrigated desert climates. The grain belt of the Midwest has the highest counts of molds, especially molds called *Alternaria* and *Hormodendrum*. Small grains such as oats and rye are common hosts for molds.

An allergist will know which molds are commonly found in a particular local area. If a person is sensitive to molds, the characteristic symptoms may correlate directly with the distribution of molds in the air at certain times of the year. Frequently, however, mold-sensitive persons will have a history of symptoms at times other than during the mold seasons. Confusion results because the offending molds are carried on pollen grains during a pollen season.

The symptoms of allergy may be aggravated during the warmer months, or there may be no coincidence between the symptoms and the seasons. An allergic person may have a positive history of reactions to molds but not experience any seasonal variation. Symptoms may be caused by molds found in the environment year-round.

Year-round (Perennial) Molds

Perennial molds, those that last throughout the entire year, are as much a problem to most allergic persons as the seasonal types that flourish in warm, humid weather. Sometimes the only indication of a mold's presence is a musty odor.

Common sources for molds are found in the "**Source Index**" under "**Molds.**"

ENVIRONMENTALS

Environmental allergens include those substances found inside homes, workplaces and schools. They may include any plant or animal substance or a product used in building or decorating. Examples of vegetable fibers that can cause allergy are cotton and flax. These fibers can cause allergy and provide a place for molds to develop and grow. Other sources are less obvious, such as horsehair in a Chinese rug or animal dander on the clothing in a closet. Environmentals also include air pollutants found in the air, insects, and house dust. The index at the back of the book lists common allergens alphabetically and describes where they can be found.

House Dust

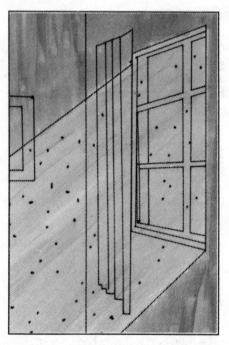

The dust that causes allergy symptoms is not the dust that blows in from outdoors. This unique dust is composed of the breakdown of plant and animal fibers in the environment. Because each home is unique in the fibers that are selected for it, house dust varies greatly from home to home. Plant fibers, such as flax and cotton, and the danders of animals, such as dogs or cats, are in furnishings and make up the main ingredients of house dust. Besides these plant and animal fibers, molds, bacteria, and food particles, the house-dust mite can also contribute to this unique substance. Because all of these materials can exist in house dust, it is difficult to determine the most common allergen. Dust mites may be the most allergenic component of dust.

The number of dust particles normally found in the environment is tremendous. A ray of light coming in a window illuminates some of the dust particles floating in the air. These visible particles will break down even more. The ultimate size may be so small that 7,000 of them could fit on the head of a pin!

The illustrations on the following page will give an idea of the relative size of some dust particles.

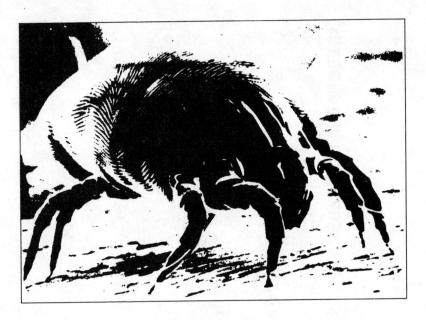

Common House Mite (Dermatophagoides Farinae) MALE

Dust mites, which are not quite visible to the unaided eye, have short lives, about 30 days. The female lays approximately one egg each day. The mites live in mattresses, carpets and upholstered furniture. Dust mites are more abundant in humid warm areas but exist throughout the world. These amazing creatures have been known to go into dormancy, if environmental conditions are not correct. The unique thing about these mites is that they live off the skin scales that humans shed. Their waste or feces is a major source of house-dust allergy.

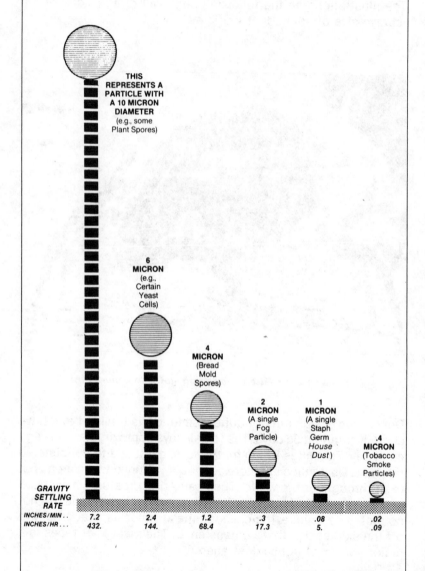

APPROXIMATE GRAVITY SETTLING RATE OF SOME COMMON INVISIBLE AIR BORNE PARTICLES *
ROOM TEMPERATE, 25° C or 70° F

THIS REPRESENTS A PARTICLE WITH A 10 MICRON DIAMETER (e.g., some Plant Spores)

6 MICRON (e.g., Certain Yeast Cells)

4 MICRON (Bread Mold Spores)

2 MICRON (A single Fog Particle)

1 MICRON (A single Staph Germ *House Dust*)

.4 MICRON (Tobacco Smoke Particles)

GRAVITY SETTLING RATE						
INCHES/MIN ..	7.2	2.4	1.2	.3	.08	.02
INCHES/HR ...	432.	144.	68.4	17.3	5.	.09

* Assume particles to be spheres of pure water at sea level in ABSOLUTELY motionless air.

INSECTS

The insect allergy that most persons have heard about is the allergy to bee venom. However, a number of other insects can also cause trouble. It is not just their stings that can produce reactions in sensitive persons. Like pollens, insects are prevalent during certain seasons. When insects swarm, carcasses and body parts can be inhaled or come into contact with the skin and cause the symptoms of allergy.

Stinging insects*, often called *Hymenoptera*, can be divided into two families. One family is the apids, which include honey bees and bumblebees. The second family, the vespids, includes yellow jackets, hornets, and wasps. Non-winged *Hymenoptera* are also included in the stinging insects. These include the fire ant and harvester ant that are found in the southern part of the United States.

* Please see illustration on following page.

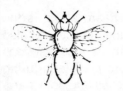

Honeybee

Honeybees   Easily recognized by their small, stocky, brown, yellow, or black bodies with a round abdomen. Probably the best-known insect, honeybees are found most frequently in artificial hives, but the colonies may be found in natural nests inside the trunks of trees, under floorboards, and in other enclosed areas. The stinger differs from that of the yellow jacket, wasp, or hornet, in that it cannot be used repeatedly (the stinging apparatus is severed from the body after the sting, the stinger is left in the skin, and the bee dies).

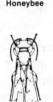

Wasp

Wasps   Black or brown with yellow or white stripes and a fusiform (tapering toward each end) abdomen. The wasp can be distinguished from the yellow jacket and the hornet by its thin waist, which joins the abdomen and the thorax. Wasps are not as excitable as the other stinging insects; they usually sting only if touched or brushed while in flight around the nest. They build their nests in trees or around shelters such as the eaves of houses or porches. The nest is usually small and contains thirty to sixty insects.

Hornet

Hornets   Black body with white markings on the thorax and abdomen. The face, excluding the top of the head, is also white. Hornets may be difficult to distinguish from yellow jackets, since they often have yellow markings. Hornets' nests are large, gray, or brown and are located in tree branches, under the eaves of houses, or against a wall, usually more than four feet above the ground. Hornets are considered the most aggressive of the major stinging insects, sometimes attacking without apparent provocation.

Yellow Jacket

Yellow Jackets   are located in the ground, often in tall grass between the walls of buildings or under stones.

Fire Ant

Fire Ants   Introduced from South America during the 1920s, fire ants are now well established in several Southern states. The venom of the fire ant differs from that of hymenoptera insects, in that it can produce severe local reactions or systemic anaphylactic reactions. The insect attacks by biting to secure itself, then inserts its stinging apparatus, which contains the venom. Highly sensitive patients with high levels of allergic antibodies against the venom of the fire ant are usually treated with immunotherapy.

Stinging Insects Illustrated

Source: **Allergy Encyclopedia**

Permission to print the following descriptions and sketches by Phil Jones has been granted by the Asthma and Allergy Foundation of America. It is from the Allergy Encyclopedia, out of print.

4

IRRITANTS— THE UNBALANCERS

The term "irritant" refers to those substances that trigger an impending allergy reaction or those substances that facilitate a reaction. Irritant sources include the weather, climate, chemicals, and physical states such as fatigue or stress. Any one of these can trigger trouble by throwing off the body's balance. Those unbalancers related to weather, climate, and chemicals are discussed in this chapter.

WEATHER AND CLIMATE

Frequently, allergic people require medical treatment whenever sudden changes in temperature, barometric pressure, or humidity occur. For example, if a cold front enters a region, allergic people who are sensitive to sharp drops in barometric pressure may find that they are more prone to respond to the allergens in their environment.

Not much can be done to control the weather, but some steps can be taken to control the climate within the environment. See Chapter Six on building.

The weather can affect the body in several ways. Low barometric pressure can cause the body tissues to soak up water from the intestines as pressure drops. Some persons complain of nasal, sinus, or joint problems during the drop. This tissue swelling may make a person feel clumsy and reduce the blood supply to the brain. Fog may depress some people or make them feel cold or less efficient. Wind can produce fatigue and dry wind will trigger upper respiratory irritation as nasal passages dry. Dry air with warm temperatures interferes with the normal moist clearing action of the membranes. The result is a reduction of secretions that rid the system of foreign matter. When the air is too moist, interference with natural evaporation from the skin and mucous membranes results. An allergic person who has any of these physical responses may have to take special precautions during particular weather conditions.

CHEMICAL IRRITANTS

This section deals with the chemicals that frequently cause adverse reactions in everyone, not just allergic people. Frequently the term "chemical sensitivity" is used to describe a reaction by some people to chemicals. Because no definite distinctions are made, or recognized, among chemical allergens, chemical sensitivity, poisons or toxins, use of this label is controversial and raises a number of questions.

Is a person susceptible because of a constitutional problem that encourages symptoms? Is the person so overwhelmed by chemical contaminants in the environment that the body reacts? Is the person failing to adapt to chemical changes in the environment? Are many chemicals toxic to all humans, and do some people become ill more easily? Are chemicals in the environment poisonous in small dosages until a point is reached at which the sensitive person becomes ill from them? Are humans slowly becoming toxic from the environment? Is there maladaptation due to illness? These questions have yet to be answered. Allergists in the United States tend to put this area of concern outside their field because of all the unanswered questions. They do recognize, however, that chemicals do unbalance the body in some way, but this process is not allergy.

The chemical environment includes outdoor air pollutants, indoor pollutants, and occupational and personal pollutants, such as cosmetics, cleaning products, water and fabric conditioners, drugs, and food additives.

AIR POLLUTION

Because it is recognized that air pollution adversely affects those who suffer from respiratory allergies, what can be done besides supporting legislation and community groups dedicated to cleaning the air? Just about nothing. Strenuous outdoor physical activities can be reduced, as many school physical education programs are doing in the larger cities. Filters made of activated charcoal or certain chemicals can be used to prevent pollutants from coming into the home, car, or office. Sensitive persons can stay indoors. Because the air pollution problems outside cannot be solved immediately, interior air pollutants must be controlled so that the interior environment can serve as a refuge or recovery area.

To effectively control the environment, the sources must be well understood. Outdoor air pollutants include industrial air pollutants, pollutants from motors that use any combustible fuel, pesticides, and tars. The following are major contributors to air pollution

1. **Hydrocarbons.** Hydrocarbons are compounds from escaped unburned fuel. This type of air pollutant is usually invisible. It is frequently called photochemical smog and is formed by the action of sunlight on nitrogen oxides and hydrocarbons. The automobile is the biggest source of this type of air pollution.

2. **Nitrogen oxides.** Nitrogen oxides form a brownish haze. Combustion of all types of fuel causes release of these compounds.

3. **Sulfur oxides.** Sulfur oxides are formed wherever coal or oil are burned.

4. **Major industrial sources.** Pulp and paper mills, petroleum refineries, smelters, inorganic chemical manufacturers, organic chemical manufacturers, production of electricity, and burning of trash are a few examples of industrial sources.

INDOOR AIR POLLUTION

With the construction of buildings that are sealed and energy efficient, exposure to pollutants inside buildings has recently become an area of concern. Some common new terms have come into the medical literature, such as "sick building syndrome," "tight building syndrome," and "building sickness." The National Institute for Occupational Safety and Health (NIOSH) has described consistent symptoms experienced by people exposed to chemicals in these buildings. Symptoms can include eye irritation, a dry scratchy throat, headache, fatigue, shortness of breath, cough, dizziness, or nausea.

Three other types of illness also have been described in the literature. The first of these is allergy — hay fever or bronchial asthma — that is aggravated by pollen, mold, dust, or other allergens that circulate inside a building's air. Allergens can accumulate in poorly ventilated offices or buildings and cause symptoms of allergy.

The second is infection. Poor ventilation in energy efficient, well-insulated buildings can permit the growth of some infectious organisms. An excellent example of this occurred several years ago when 221 people who were attending an American Legion convention in Philadelphia became seriously ill and 31 of them died. The lethal organism which caused this illness was eventually traced to the water spray found within the hotel's cooling tower.

Irritation of the skin and eyes is the last type of illness that can be attributed to buildings with poor air circulation. In addition, some factories may have particles in the air that, while not causing immediate symptoms, may cause serious health problems after prolonged exposure. These particles include fiberglass and asbestos.

COMMON OFFICE EXPOSURES

PHOTOCOPYING MACHINES
FIBERS
ADHESIVES
CLEANING AGENTS
CORRECTION FLUID
RUBBER CEMENT
CARBONLESS CARBON PAPER
VENTILATION SYSTEM THAT MOVES AIR
THROUGHOUT BUILDING

Potentially hazardous chemicals that can spread through ventilation systems can be found in air fresheners, adhesives, cleaning solvents, off-gases,* copying machines, fire retardants and other maintenance fluids or chemicals used in the office or home environment. Thus the products used to build, decorate, and clean homes to enhance lifestyle can then become sources for illness. These sources for pollution in the interior environment frequently have warning labels, but we tend to use these products carelessly.

* See Chapter Six for description of "off-gassing"

The sources that require the most awareness include combustion products; tobacco smoke; consumer products, such as household cleaning or cosmetic products; organic chemicals; pesticides; particulates or solid particles in the air; and formaldehyde. Other sources that may have a detrimental effect but are not as common include asbestos, lead, radon, air ions, nonionizing radiation, plastic pipe for potable water, and light and noise pollution. This is a long list, and it is only recently that these sources have been publicized as being potentially harmful. As a result, they are in the environment because no one knew better.

In 1982, the California Department of Consumer Affairs published the "Compendium on Indoor Pollution" that included some of the following information on pollutants that can result in physical symptoms.

Formaldehyde

The use of formaldehyde in insulation and other building materials has resulted in the coining of the new medical term "mobile home syndrome." This syndrome came to light when the occupants of mobile homes began developing mysterious illnesses. Investigation eventually revealed that urea formaldehyde foam insulation and particle board containing a urea formaldehyde resin adhesive, both of which were used extensively in the construction of mobile homes, were associated with this illness. Foam insulation was also injected into the sidewalls of conventional homes until around 1977 when other insulation products became widely used.

Formaldehyde is used in a number of other consumer products. People who are sensitive to formaldehyde must be alert to the fact that it is used in some textiles, as well as in plywood, carpeting and molded plastics. In addition, tobacco smoke, gas stoves, wood stoves and kerosene space heaters all emit formaldehyde. The California report suggests reducing the emissions from these sources by ventilating the area to clean the air.

GUIDELINES FOR CONTROLLING FORMALDEHYDE SOURCES

- Remove the formaldehyde source if possible.
- Cover walls with a nonporous material and seal electrical or plumbing outlets.
- Keep windows open with cross ventilation as much as possible.
- Move.

Tobacco Smoke

In 1986, the Surgeon General's report made strong statements about the detrimental effects that smoking had on nonsmokers. Smoking is more than a personal choice. The health hazards of passive smoking or sidestream smoke that the nonsmoker experiences are well documented. Prolonged exposure is a health hazard not only for infants, children, pregnant women, the elderly and people with cardiovascular or pulmonary disease, but for healthy people as well. It is obvious that elimination of tobacco smoke from the environment is a benefit to all.

SMOKING GUIDELINES

✦ A smoker in one area of a home or office can contaminate the entire building. Fine particles move throughout and stay suspended in the air for hours. See chart in Chapter Six on the length of time particles can stay in the air.

✦ If "NO SMOKING" rules cannot be enforced, select a filter system for the air conditioning system or for a room that can be isolated from the rest of the building's air supply. Purchase the appropriate filter type and make certain enough air is circulated to filter the fine particles out of the air.

✦ Call your local American Lung Association for "NO SMOKING" signs, stop smoking programs and for further information.

Combustion Products

Because the home is closed, exposure to the byproducts of combustion can be many times higher than outdoors. These gases — nitrogen dioxide and carbon monoxide — can be produced inside the home by heating equipment that uses gas, oil, kerosene or wood; gas water heaters and clothes dryers; tobacco smoke; and automobile exhaust from an attached garage. Therefore, homes must be designed carefully to ventilate these fumes. Hood fans, flues, windows, or doors can help to dispose of gases. Keeping equipment running efficiently and ventilating the interior air are key ways to control exposure to the byproducts of combustion.

Organic Chemicals

Chemicals are a source for health hazards in a number of indoor environments. These chemicals may be found in structural or decorative materials; cleaning agents; or the products used for indoor activities such as cooking, hobbies, paint stripping, and many others.

Newer buildings have a higher concentration of chemicals. It takes time for these chemicals to disappear from the air. In new office buildings, it can take up to six months before chemicals are substantially cleaned from the air.

Chemicals and some equipment in the workplace expose the user to health problems. Again, these may not cause the symptoms of allergy; however, they throw the body's balance into jeopardy. Some examples are solvents used to operate equipment, especially copying machines and printing equipment. Cleaning compounds such as detergents used for synthetic carpets and furniture can leave a residue that can later be inhaled if it has not been cleaned out of the fibers.

Regardless of where chemicals are found — whether in the home, workplace or school — more definite information about how to detect toxic levels is needed. Research on the subject, and services that can detect the presence of potentially harmful chemicals are limited at this time. The best indicator of whether a harmful chemical is present in any particular area is an individual's reaction when in that environment. If someone goes into an environment and begins to experience physical symptoms, they should carefully assess the situation to determine if there is something present in the environment that is not found in places where they ordinarily spend their time. For example: Are they in a newly constructed building? Is there equipment, such as a copying machine, in the area? What kinds of decorative materials are in the room? Has the carpeting and/or furniture been recently shampooed? Is air from another part of the building coming into the area? If a suspected problem cannot be remedied easily, they can choose to avoid that area.

Pesticides

Insecticides have so many uses that the potential for exposure is very great. In nearly 90 percent of households, pesticides are used inside the home, in the garden, or on lawns. Some pesticides do not break down quickly; consequently, the chemicals remain active for years. Outdoor chemicals can get indoors on clothing and through open windows and doors. Pesticides are not restricted to killing pests listed on the label. To some degree, they affect every living thing.

The chemicals used by a professional insecticide service can expose anyone who is in the area at the time of application, as well as those who enter the area for a given time afterwards. The length of time depends upon the chemicals used and the time it takes for those particular chemicals to break down to a harmless state. Mothballs, slow-release insect strips and flea collars can also result in exposure to potentially harmful chemicals. In addition, the food supply may be exposed to numerous pesticides that are very difficult to trace or identify. Unfortunately, even if a company claims there is not a toxic exposure to be concerned about, sensitive people need to be aware that there are not well-documented guidelines for toxic levels of these types of chemicals for the length of time they may remain toxic. There are only guidelines for those individuals who have documented evidence of a chemical's harmful effect on their health.

Because the home interior is protected from the wind and sun's ultraviolet light, the breakdown of insecticides can take longer than for products used outdoors. For this reason, reapplication of an insecticide may unnecessarily result in a buildup of chemicals. Chlordane, for example, can remain active where it has been applied for 20 years or longer.

GUIDELINES FOR CONTROL OF INTERIOR POLLUTION SOURCES

For people who have allergies, products that disperse into the air, emit strong odors, or leave a residue are potential sources for allergic symptoms. Even if a person is not specifically allergic to the materials or products used in the environment, these products may serve as a source of irritatin to unbalance the person's physical condition. For this reason we have provided some guidelines to avoid these chemicals.

GUIDELINES FOR USING CLEANING PRODUCTS IN THE HOME

✦ Avoid all aerosols in the home. Substitute liquid or dry forms of the same product.

✦ For odor control, clean the source producing the odor or ventilate the area. Deodorants "mask" odors; they do not eliminate them.

✦ Use unscented cosmetic and toiletry products.

✦ Avoid pesticides. Use mechanical or natural means for control, such as electric traps, fly swatters, or removal of the source that attracts insects or animals. Learn about herbs and insects that eliminate annoying insects. Most gardening books explain methods of insect control that use nontoxic products.

✦ Avoid the use of air fresheners, adhesives, cleaning solvents, aerosols and strong-scented cleaning products in the home or office without ventilation from outside. Use a solution of borax and water to disinfect.

✦ Wear rubber gloves when applying furniture cleaners or floor polishes.

✦ Use nontoxic cleaning products such as:
  • Baking soda
  • Salt
  • Distilled white vinegar
  • Lemon juice
  • Trisodium phosphate (TSP)
  • Borax

✦ Use vinegar in water for cleaning whenever possible rather than all the elaborate compounds now sold. Use a 50/50 solution for a spray bottle.

✦ Use baking soda, dissolved with water, for cleaning coffee pots, chrome, copper, and tile.

— CONTINUED —

✦ As an alternative to oven cleaners, use ammonia or baking soda. Sprinkle on dry soda, let stand for five minutes, then wipe with a damp cloth. Ammonia placed in a non-aluminum dish filled with water and left overnight in the oven is another alternative.

✦ Use nontoxic and biodegradable soaps. In areas with hard water use water softeners such as Calgon or baking soda.

✦ Instead of furniture cleaners, use carnauba wax mixed with mineral oil (one tablespoon wax into two cups of oil) or make your own lemon oil (a teaspoon of lemon oil into a pint of mineral oil).

✦ To make a mold and mildew cleaner, mix borax and water (1 tsp to 1 qt.), vinegar and water (1 tsp. to 1 qt.) in a spray bottle. The borax can be sprayed on and left to dry under sinks or damp cabinets.

✦ Be aware that labels on products are not consistent. Poison labeling may not be clear or bold enough to be noticed. The amount of a product's inert contents or its propellant may not be listed.

GUIDELINES FOR VENTILATING AND FILTERING AIR

✦ Check and clean refrigeration equipment once a year to be sure that the air intake and the exhaust system are working correctly. The interior working parts can harbor dust, bacteria and molds.

✦ Properly maintain flues and chimneys to prevent fumes from going down into the home.

✦ Gas burners should burn with a blue flame. An orange flame or flickering flames are indicators that the burner needs cleaning.

— CONTINUED —

- ✦ Poke a wood fire so it will burn down before going to bed. When burning wood, be sure there is an open source of fresh air.
- ✦ If new carpet has been installed, ventilate the home with outside air for several days. Very sensitive people may have to stay out of the home for a week or more.
- ✦ New buildings or newly redecorated buildings should have more than the usual amount of ventilation from outside for several months. Heat will also speed up the "off-gassing" process.
- ✦ Utilize exhaust fans while cooking or using any chemicals, especially glues.
- ✦ Avoid stove fans that recirculate air rather than exhaust it out of the home.
- ✦ Follow current federal information for testing and eliminating radon exposure.

DRUGS AND MEDICINES

Prescription and nonprescription medications may affect people in one or several ways. Allergic reactions can occur to the drug itself, to the contents of the capsule, to the filler or to the syrup, or to preservatives in the medication.

Many of the frequently used over-the-counter (nonprescription) drugs, as well as the drugs prescribed by the physician, can cause symptoms. The following list gives an idea of the wide distribution of foods and chemicals used in the drug industry:

mint	glycerin	cherry	cocoa butter
coconut	vitamins	alcohol	saccharin
chocolate	cane suger	arrowroot	tapioca
rice	wheat	yeast	citrus
pork	beef	starch	acacia
potato	lactose	sucrose	corn
egg	peanut oil		

FIBER FINISHES

As if polluted air, foods, drugs, and cosmetics were not enough to worry about, the finishes on fabrics must be considered. These finishes are frequent causes of physical symptoms. Some can be washed out; others are a permanent part of the fiber. Many people blame some of the new synthetic fibers for allergy symptoms when it is really the fiber finish that causes the trouble. Some of the synthetic fibers do not breathe, and the skin is irritated by warmth. If new clothing or bedding is washed and thoroughly rinsed before being put to use, many allergy symptoms could be avoided.

Some of the finishes are as follows:

FINISH	INFORMATION
✓ Formaldehyde *	Used to treat a majority of fabrics to give fresh new finish; produces maximum crush-resistance with minimum stiffening.
✓ Plasticized starch	Usually found on 100 percent cotton.
✓ DDT	Found in professionally cleaned garments, dry cleaning fluids, and indoor/outdoor carpet fibers.
✓ Soap residue. *	Found on anything washed and not well-rinsed, especially in hard water.
✓ Fabric softeners *	Remains in the fiber and builds up a residue.
✓ Starch *	Remains in the fiber and builds up a residue.
✓ Dyes	Can be chemical dyes or natural from plants.

* Can be washed out of the fabric.

GUIDELINES
FOR SUBSTITUTING FINISHES
OR APPLYING FINISHES

The following are suggestions for applying
fabric finishes or can be used as substitutes:

✦ Use a paint brush or home spray to waterproof
   fabric with liquid fabric finishes.

✦ Apply fabric finishes outdoors.
   Eliminate static cling by keeping the air
   humidified, or spray the fabric with a mister.

✦ Wear gloves and work in a ventilated space with
   outdoor air to apply spot removers.

✦ Use laundry soda in the rinse cycle to remove
   residues.

✦ Wash all new fabrics before wearing or using
   them.

You have now developed an awareness of allergens and
pollutants that upset balance outside your body. In the later
chapters, you will learn ways to control exposure to allergens
and pollutants in building, decorating, or cleaning a home. At
this point, the focus will switch to balancing components within
our bodies.

5

✦

LIFESTYLE—
A BALANCING
ACT

ANALYZING YOUR LIFESTYLE

Often, an allergic person's lifestyle is like a roller coaster. The ups and downs experienced from day to day, feeling well one day and ill the next, can make life very unpredictable. If this is true for you, perhaps it is time to take a close look at your total lifestyle and become aware of elements in your life that affect your ability to function effectively.

Bearing in mind the elements in your lifestyle that must be in balance for you to achieve a condition of total positive health, you can begin to set up a lifestyle priority list. Such a list should include the following basic components:

1• Thoroughly examine your exposures to allergens. Determine where you spend most of your time and what exposures are present. Eliminate allergenic sources that exist in your home. It has been found that the amount of relief from symptoms is directly proportional to how thoroughly you succeed in eliminating the allergens from your home enviornment.

2• Determine what physical conditions in the environment such as temperature or weather changes affect the pattern of your symptoms. Determine which irritants such as smoke and air pollutants affect you and devise ways to reduce your exposure to those factors.

3• Determine the condition of your body. Review your dietary habits, your exercise routines, the balance between your work and play times, and the proper use of medications. Review your personal health risk factors at the end of the chapter.

4• Assess the emotional part of your life. Determine which stresses exist in your life and what you are going to do about them. Determine how positive you are in your approach to life, your values, your feelings about yourself and your body, and whether or not you are satisfied with your spiritual development.

In setting up your priority list, you may wish to refer to the assessment included in Chapter Two.

Stress

Your lifestyle is a matter of personal choice; however, you may get into a pattern that is not in your best interest. One of these patterns is unhealthy stress. Stress plays such a major role in health in our culture that it warrants special attention. Stress over the years may manifest itself as high blood pressure, a chronic illness, heart disease or a host of health complaints. It is interesting to note that 30 percent of our nation's population has 70 percent of the illnesses. These persons frequently have multiple illnesses, especially those illnesses related to thoughts and feelings. It is impossible to tell exactly how stress plays its role in contributing to illness. However, persons who are adept at coping with stress have a lower chance of becoming ill. Those who cope well are usually not part of the 30 percent of the population who experience most of the illnesses.

To give you an idea of your chances of becoming ill from stress, take the following Life Events Stress Test developed by Dr. Rahe.

After you have taken this test, review your score. If you scored below 150, you have a 10 percent chance of having a significant illness. If you scored between 150 and 300 you have a 50 percent chance. A score higher than 300 indicates you have a 90 percent chance of being hospitalized or having a significant illness. Since Drs. Holmes and Rahe developed this test, the degree of stress may have changed over time. For example, a $10,000 mortgage or loan should probably be many thousands more. Nevertheless, the test gives you a perspective that change causes stress; some changes are more stressful than others.

The fact that most of these life events do not occur entirely by chance means you can have some control over your future. You can predict life events and their outcomes to some degree and plan to manage life changes by adjusting your financial status, your pace in life, and so on. The point to remember is that if you "plan" change in your life, you can avoid getting into the high probability range for illness.

What is Stress?

Stress is difficult to define. It can be compared to body temperature. Everyone has a normal body temperature. Usually, if it rises above 98.6 degrees Fahrenheit, a person is thought to be ill. Stress can be thought of as such a continuum as well. If you have no stress, you are dead, just as you are dead without temperature. If you think of a scale of 0 to 100 with 0 being death and 100 being extreme distress, you can begin to find your best level of functioning. For instance, humans need some degree of stress to feel motivated and to grow. If stress falls below that level, persons become unmotivated and probably depressed.

On such an arbitrary scale, a person can function well between 40 and 70. Once above or below this range, illness can result. Stress carries us toward life's accomplishments. Without it, we do not grow. At each end of the continuum, constant high or low stress makes a person ill. The ideal course is to maintain a

HOW CLOSE TO THE EDGE ARE YOU?

At the University of Washington Medical School in Seattle, Drs. Thomas H. Holmes and Richard H. Rahe devised a "Social Readjustment Rating Scale" test, which lists forty-two common life changes in the order in which they found them to be important as precursors of illness.

1• Death of spouse .... 100 _____
2• Divorce .... 73 _____
3• Marital separation .... 65 _____
4• Jail term .... 63 _____
5• Death of close
   family member .... 63 _____
6• Personal injury
   or illness .... 53 _____
7• Marriage .... 50 _____
8• Fired from work .... 47 _____
9• Marital reconciliation.. 45 _____
10• Retirement .... 45 _____
11• Change in family
    member's health .... 44 _____
12• Pregnancy .... 40 _____
13• Sex difficulties .... 39 _____
14• Addition to family .... 39 _____
15• Business
    readjustment .... 39 _____
16• Change in
    financial status .... 38 _____
17• Death of close friend.. 37 _____
18• Change in number of
    marital arguments .... 35 _____
19• Mortgage or loan
    over $10,000 .... 31 _____
20• Foreclosure of
    mortgage or loan .... 30 _____
21• Change in work
    responsibilities .... 29 _____
22• Son or daughter
    leaving home .... 29 _____
23• Trouble with in-laws .... 29 _____

24• Outstanding personal
    achievement .... 28 _____
25• Spouse begins or
    starts work .... 26 _____
26• Starting or finishing
    school .... 26 _____
27• Change in living
    conditions .... 25 _____
28• Revision of
    personal habits .... 24 _____
29• Trouble with boss .... 23 _____
30• Change in work hours,
    conditions .... 20 _____
31• Change in residence... 20 _____
32• Change in schools ...... 20 _____
33• Change in
    recreational habits ...... 19 _____
34• Change in
    church activities .... 19 _____
35• Change in
    social activities .... 18 _____
36• Mortgage or loan
    under $10,000 .... 18 _____
37• Change in
    sleeping habits .... 16 _____
38• Change in number
    of family gatherings.... 15 _____
39• Change in eating habits 15 _____
40• Vacation .... 13 _____
41• Christmas season .... 12 _____
42• Minor violation of law. 11 _____

TOTAL _____

balance between the two ends. This ideal range results from a total positive lifestyle: a balance of good nutrition, exercise, a positive attitude toward life, and effective coping skills to control negative stress.

Stress A Continuum

Distress		Distress
Death		Extreme Upset
0 10 20 30	40 50 60 70	80 90 100
Dysfunction		Dysfunction
Depression	Growing	Hypertension
Unmotivated	Motivated	Physical
Inactive	Feeling of Well Being	Symptoms

Stress Scale

How do you know if you have effective coping skills? The following questionnaire lists 10 questions so you can assess how you may react in different situations.

SITUATIONAL QUESTIONNAIRE

Instructions: For each item, please rate the degree to which the incident described by the item would upset you by using the following scale:

1 • You don't react

2 • You say *Oh well!!*

3 • You display a moderate degree of upset that quickly passes

4 • You say something obscene and get physically upset

5 • You have a temper tantrum

Try to imagine the incident actually happening to you, and then indicate the extent to which it would have made you upset.

_____ ① You are waiting to be served at a restaurant. Fifteen minutes have gone by, and you still have not even received a menu.

_____ ② You unpack an appliance that you have just bought, plug it in, and discover that it does not work.

_____ ③ You are driving to pick up a friend at the airport and are forced to wait for a long freight train. You will be late.

_____ ④ Your car is stalled at a traffic light, and the guy behind you keeps blowing his horn.

_____ ⑤ You are being criticized in front of others for something that you have done.

_____ ⑥ You have had a busy day, and the person you live with starts to complain about how you forgot to do something that you agreed to do.

_____ ⑦ You are trying to discuss something important with your mate or partner who is not giving you a chance to express your feelings.

_____ ⑧ You are having an intense discussion with someone and another person interrupts.

⑨ You use 20 cents to make a phone call, but you are disconnected before you finish dialing. You only have dollar bills.

_____ ⑩ In a hurry to get somewhere, you tear a good pair of slacks on a sharp object.

_____ ◄ **TOTAL SCORE**

Once you have finished the questions, add up the points in the column. If you have a score less than 10, you interpret stress calmly or passively. A score of 10 to 20 is a healthy range, and more than 20 may indicate that you interpret stress in a unhealthy way. Fill in your score on the Risk Profile at the end of the chapter.

If you scored less than 10, you may be using healthy coping habits or unhealthy ones, depending on how you "feel." If you reacted in a calm manner and you are aware you feel upset, you probably are reacting in a healthy manner if you act on the situation in a positive manner. If you do not feel anything, you are probably suppressing your feelings. If so, you are reacting passively, and this can lead to illness. Be aware of how your body reacts to stress. See the list of some of the common physical responses.

INDICATORS OF STRESS

Physiological	Behavioral	Intellectual Cues
• General irritability	• Depression	• Forgetfulness
• Over-excited	• Impulsive Behavior	• Preoccupation
• Pounding of the heart	• Emotional instability	• Reviewing an event
• Dryness of the throat and mouth	• Overpowering urge to cry, run or retreat	over and over in your head
• Feelings of weakness	• Feelings of unreality	• Mathematical or
• Dizziness	• Predilection to become	grammatical errors
• Trembling	fatigued or loss of zest	• Errors in judging space
• Nervous Tics	• Floating anxiety	• Memory blocks
• Tendency to be easily startled by small sounds	(intermittent feelings of anxiety without apparent reason)	• Diminished fantasy life
• Inability to sit still	• High-pitched laugh	• Lack of concentration
• Sweating	• Insomnia	• Reduction in interest
• Frequent need to urinate	• Stuttering or other speech difficulty	• Lack of attention to details
• Frequent need to defecate	• Grinding of teeth	• Past-oriented rather than present-
• Diarrhea	• Increased smoking	or future-oriented
• Nausea	• Increased use of prescribed or	• Lack of awareness of external stimuli
• Pain in the neck or lower back	unprescribed drugs	• Reduction in creativity
• Loss of or excessive appetite	• Increased use of alcohol	• Diminished productivity
• Sweaty palms	• Nightmares	
• Susceptibility to minor illness	• Accident proneness	
	• Diminished initiative	
	• Tendency to blame others	

Over the years persons learn to respond in particular patterns. Some of these patterns may be unhealthy for you or for those around you. If you examine how your pattern has developed, you can better see how you can control your response to undesirable stress.

For example, a stressful event is one that is perceived as stressful. This perception depends on past experiences and how you reacted. The stressful event also is conditioned by your state of health — the diet you eat, your physical condition, your inherited traits, your age, and your sex. If you learned to react in a aggressive way, you will continue to react in that manner until you decide to work on changing.

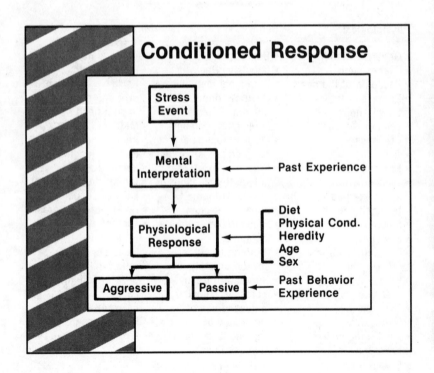

Conditioned Response

If you find that your response pattern is not healthy, there are some alternatives. You can begin to control your reactions to negative stress. Look at the "**Alternatives**" chart and review how you react. You can see that you have two immediate choices; healthy or unhealthy ways to respond. If you responded in an unhealthy manner, you still have the opportunity to make a choice to make the situation healthy. You can use a stress reduction technique to eliminate the stress from your body. Some of these techniques are described later.

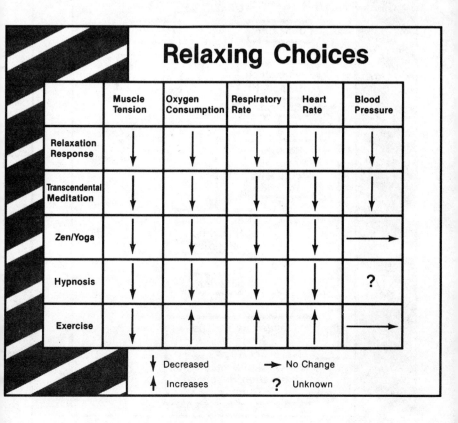

Relaxing Choices

	Muscle Tension	Oxygen Consumption	Respiratory Rate	Heart Rate	Blood Pressure
Relaxation Response	↓	↓	↓	↓	↓
Transcendental Meditation	↓	↓	↓	↓	↓
Zen/Yoga	↓	↓	↓	↓	→
Hypnosis	↓	↓	↓	↓	?
Exercise	↓	↑	↑	↑	→

↓ Decreased   → No Change
↑ Increases   ? Unknown

Body's Response to Different Methods of Relaxation

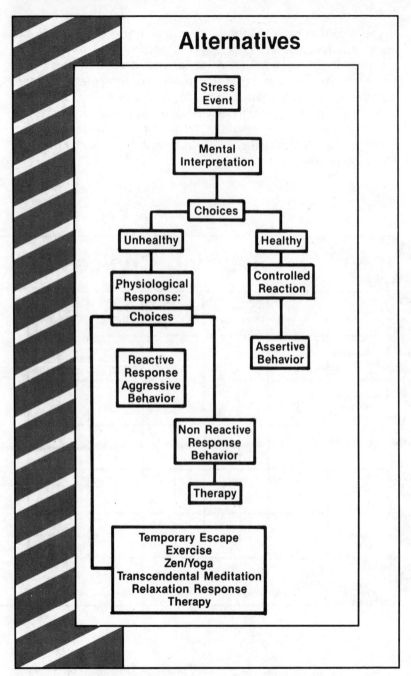

Healthy and Unhealthy Responses to Stressful Events

✦

INSTRUCTIONS TO ELICIT
THE RELAXATION RESPONSE

There are many variations to relaxation as seen on the graphic "**Relaxing Choices.**" Some include imaging, stretching, biofeedback and others. The following steps outline the basic technique.

1• Sit quietly in a comfortable position.

2• Close your eyes.

3• Beginning at your feet and progressing up to your face, deeply relax all your muscles. Keep them relaxed.

4• Breathe through your nose. Become aware of your breathing. As you breathe out, say the word "one" silently to yourself. Continue the pattern: breathe in ... out, "one," in out, "one," and so on. Breathe easily and naturally.

5• Continue for 10-20 minutes. You may open your eyes to check the time, but do not use an alarm. When you finish, sit quietly for a few minutes, first with your eyes closed and later with you eyes opened. Do not stand up for a few minutes.

6• Do not worry about whether you are successful in achieving a deep level of relaxation. Maintain a passive attitude and permit relaxation to occur at its own pace. When distracting thoughts occur, try to ignore them by not dwelling on them and return to repeating "one." With practice, the response should come with little effort. Practice the technique once or twice daily but not within two hours after any meal, since the digestive processes seem to interfere with eliciting the relaxation response.

RX GUIDELINES
FOR TOTAL POSITIVE HEALTH

Guidelines for total positive health might include the following 10 steps.

✦ Constantly assess the satisfactions of life around you.
   - Are you having fun?
   - How do you look?
     Is your skin, posture, body language energetic, vibrant and lively looking?
   - How do you feel?
   - Are you causing stress in those around you?

✦ Develop an attitude that if you cannot change a situation, then you will love it. You resolve stress in this way.

✦ Eat what makes you feel good.

✦ Relax. Vacation and time out are a necessity.

✦ Sleep. Program yourself in a positive way before you go to sleep.

✦ Fill in the following Risk Factor Probability Profile and see if your risks are high, medium, or low. You can set goals to reduce those risks that are on the high side.

✦ Take note of your dreams and work through them.

✦ Like yourself.

✦ Take sick leave from work when you feel like you are at your limit mentally or physically.

✦ Check and assess changes in your physical condition that you may not be aware of by taking frequent health-risk assessment.

RISK FACTOR PROFILE

Circle the box that fits you

Primary Factors	HIGH RISK	MEDIUM RISK	LOW RISK
Tobacco Consumption	1+ Pack/Day	Less than 1 Pack/Day	None
Serum Cholesterol	+ 230 Mg	180-230 Mg	Less than 180 Mg
Blood Pressure	Above 120/80		120/80 Or Less
Family History Of Heart Attack Or Strokes	Yes		No

Secondary Factors	HIGH RISK	MEDIUM RISK	LOW RISK
Diabetes	Yes		No
Physical Exercise	None	Walk, Use Stairs	Aerobic exer. at least 3x/wk for 30 min or longer
Serum Triglycerides	Elevated	Borderline Elevation	Normal

Stress Factors	HIGH RISK	MEDIUM RISK	LOW RISK
Alcohol Consumption	+ 12 Drinks Per Week	8-12 Drinks/Week	0-7 Drinks
Job Stress	High	Some Stress	Low Stress
Personal Or Family Stress	High	Some Stress	Low Stress

Allergy Factors	HIGH RISK	MEDIUM RISK	LOW RISK
Follow Prescriptions and/or Take Allergy Shots As Directed	No	Usually	Yes
Positive Environment Control Of Bedroom	No	Some	Yes
Make An Effort To Avoid Exterior/Interior Air Pollutants	No	Some	Yes
Aware Of Causes For Allergy And Avoid Sources	No	Some	Yes

If you tend to be a passive nonreactor, you have the highest pro-bability of becoming ill because of the way you respond to life's events. Because you have spent a lifetime holding in your feel-ings, changing that pattern may require psychological therapy. If you do not have psychosomatic illness or frequent illness but tend to react in a passive way, a group therapy situation can help you see alternatives in your lifestyle.

In summary , you have many choices in coping with stress. You do not have to keep repeating the same old, unrewarding patterns. Awareness of those choices, a new philosophy that stress is good for you, and the idea that you have the power to keep stress under control are the first steps toward self-improvement.

6

BUILDING OR REMODELING A HOME

For the allergic person, exposures to allergens must be considered when building or remodeling a home. Depending upon the design, the use of certain building materials and treatment or maintenance of those materials can result in an exposure to allergens. Chapter Two presented the notion that a person's lifestyle involves the interplay of many factors. The balanced interplay of these factors governs the control of allergic symptoms. Exposures to pollens, molds, and environmentals in their natural occurrence in the environment have been discussed. However, sources of exposures that may inadvertently be brought into the environment and may throw balance off have not been covered. These include exposure to air pollutants that may be hazardous to health but that remain relatively difficult to document. Exposure to pollutants inside the home is becoming an area of concern, especially as builders produce homes that are sealed and energy efficient. Evidence is accumulating that organic chemicals build up in these efficient environments and may actually be toxic to the occupants. This is not allergy per se but a hazardous exposure that throws off the body's balance. New buildings are especially prone to this problem.

Off-gassing is a term used to explain the drying process that takes place as new building materials are put into a home. This off-gassing continues for weeks or months, depending upon the materials used. One person may feel ill soon after entering a new building and another may not. For some people, there is an obvious odor to the chemicals; however, others cannot detect it. It is the organic solvents used in new building materials that become this source of indoor pollution. Ventilation of these newly refurbished or constructed areas can reduce the off-gassing exposure.

If a newly constructed building is left vacant for a period of time so that many of these organic compounds can volatize and ventilate into the atmosphere before anyone occupies the building, illnesses are eliminated. A freshly painted room can be aired before you move into it, or new furniture, especially furniture made from pressboard or plastics, can be aired in a garage or storage area before it is placed inside the home. Obviously, if a home is being remodeled or redecorated, some consideration must be made as to the potential exposures to off-gassing. Information about the type and rate of emission among various materials is available; however, little research has been done on the characteristics of the materials under different circumstances. The best guideline is to make sure that there is extra ventilation and heat during the early weeks after installation of new products. This includes decorative products, such as window coverings, flooring, and carpeting.

Building or moving to another home is a major decision for the allergic person. It is most important to discuss the move with the physician. Most allergy problems are moved along with the furnishings, and it can be very disappointing to find that an ideally constructed home is not so ideal.

The person who moves to the desert from a colder climate in hopes of improving health may be surprised to find that allergy symptoms now occur year-round instead of just in the spring. The Sunbelt climate produces pollens all year. The larger cities in the desert have just as much air pollution as their counterparts in the cooler climates.

Your physician can indicate local areas that would be more desirable for your particular allergy problems. For example, if you suffer from weed pollen allergy, you may not do well in the country. If you suffer from mold allergy, you may not do well near the ocean. Or the pollutants of industry may affect you if the wind blows from the industrial source.

Sometimes a patient will make a long-distance move and feel absolutely great for about two years, just long enough to acquire new allergies. As a rule, it is best to stay where you are and remedy the problems as best you can. Some situations, of course, do warrant a move if the allergy is to improve.

SELECTION OF THE HOME SITE

Winds

Survey the prevailing wind direction with great care. The proposed home site should not be in the prevailing wind from industrial areas, freeways, high-density airports, fire-fighting training centers, marshlands, agriculture or farming areas that carry air pollutants, pollens, or molds.

Climate

A home site that is near water should usually be avoided. The higher humidity leads to problems with molds and mildew. Areas near marshlands, open drainage ditches, and stagnant water holes are to be avoided. Damp areas such as these tend to be foggy more often than other nearby areas. An exception would be a location that has steady off-shore breezes resulting in a lower humidity. About 5 to 10 miles inland from large bodies of water is a reasonable distance for avoiding fog and mildew problems. A person with only pollen allergy may benefit from a homesite near water where pollens tend to settle out of the air because of the higher humidity.

Terrain

Canyon sites harbor many weeds and insects that may cause allergy symptoms. Heavy concentrations of vegetation, such as tree groves, should be avoided. The vegetation results in an increase in pollens, molds, and insects. Some valley sites are poor because of temperature inversion; cooler air is trapped in the valley by warm upper air. Temperature inversions are responsible for very heavy air pollution because the polluted air cannot blow away. Hilltops, on the other hand, can be just as detrimental if the site is in the path of the prevailing polluted winds. The side of the hill away from the wind is the preferred building site.

Air Pollution

The dangers of air pollution should be of primary concern. Contact the air pollution control source in your community for details on what areas are the least polluted. If this information is not available, carefully map out your prospective home and indicate wind patterns, then look to see what major pollutant sources may blow into this area.

Elevation

Persons with breathing restrictions have difficulty at higher altitudes; however, the higher altitudes often have limited levels of pollutants. There does not appear to be any particular advantage to sea level versus other altitudes for allergic people.

PLANNING AND CONSTRUCTION

Some Design Considerations

Once a home's location has been selected, the design to be used should encompass controlling the interior climate, eliminating common allergens, and using building materials that are allergen-free and easy to maintain.

While exterior materials used on the home are primarily a matter of personal preference, it is helpful to remember that the more maintenance these materials require, the greater the chances are for exposure to allergens and health hazards. For example, brick, plastic gutters and a tile roof require little maintenance. If, however, the home has wood gutters, stained wood siding, and a tar or shake roof, the potential for exposures is obviously greater because these surfaces require frequent maintenance.

A properly built home should prevent pests from entering, should have plenty of light and ventilation to eliminate molds, and should have an indoor climate that remains constant. The air should be clean, and the humidity should be maintained between 40 and 50 percent. Adherence to these requirements, which requires careful selection of interior construction materials and interior decoration, can make the difference between a miserable and pleasant environment.

Building In Moisture Control

Drainage away from the home is important; therefore, gutters or roof slopes should be designed to carry water away from the home. The ground around the home should also slope away so that water cannot accumulate near the foundation.

In recent years, contractors have put plastic sheeting beneath cement foundations to stop moisture from traveling through the cement to the home interior. For homes that do not have such a moisture barrier, water sealers can be applied to the interior surface to stop it there.

In homes constructed with a crawl space beneath the flooring, moisture can be a problem unless the underside of the home is sealed with roofing paper or a plastic. Basement walls are notorious for moisture problems. A water sealer or water-sealing paint should be applied before these surfaces are covered with decorative materials or paneling. In some cases, a layer of insulation also may be necessary. Exterior draining should be checked to make certain exterior basement walls are not collecting water and that water is draining away from the home.

Exterior Climate Control

The design of the home may dictate the type of climate the home may have. For example, in an A-frame home, it is very difficult to control the interior climate because heat rises, leaving the downstairs cold and drafty. Air must be circulated in some way to equalize the temperature. The home with a beam ceiling that follows the roofline becomes very expensive to heat and cool because it has so many more cubic feet of air to control. A home built of cement blocks becomes damp and uncomfortable during rainy weather if it is not insulated or sealed against moisture.

In cold and very warm climates, glass that is not double-paned can result in drafts and expensive heating and cooling costs. Climate problems that result from glass can be prevented in a number of ways during the design phase of building a home. Tinted glass, a vine-covered trellis on the exterior of the home, or deep inset windows can reduce unnecessary sunlight. Storm windows can be added during the winter.

Insulation is probably the single most important aspect of protection against weather. Poorly insulated walls are cold in the winter, and occupants of a home feel chilly and uncomfortable no matter how much the air may be heated. Intense summer heat can raise the roof temperature to 160 degrees Fahrenheit, resulting in heat transfer to the walls and the interior of the home. Full insulation is advised for good control. This includes insulating the ceilings, floor (if the home is above ground), and walls. When insulation is installed, vapor barriers are added to provide some ventilation. The type of insulation must be selected with care. For example, fiberglass insulation can be hazardous to the skin and respiratory tract if any of it is open to the home interior. This includes attics where heating systems can draw air that contains fine particles of glass into the home. Some insulation can produce the off-gassing discussed earlier. Insulation such as wool that can harbor insects or moisture should be avoided. Special design changes may be necessary to avoid these exposures.

Windows selected for the home should be as maintenance-free as possible. Aluminum frames with no sills are ideal but may not be your preference. If you want wood frame windows with sills, make sure that the finish is lasting and will not require frequent painting. Moisture problems from windows dripping on sills or down walls can be eliminated by using double-paned windows. Solar heat is a consideration in some locations. If a solarium is chosen to collect heat, plants used to decorate the area may produce molds in the soil that will be carried throughout the home. But in general, solar heat is a good clean alternative to forced air heating systems.

Allergic persons can be irritated by odorous sealers, coating, stains, and paints that may be used in the building of a home. By using synthetic or water-based products, some of the irritants can be reduced. The following coatings are recommended for interior and exterior use because they do not appear to give off gases once they are dry.

- Latex vinyl or acrylic paints
- Latex enamels
- Silicone
- Stained wood coated with clear silicone or polyurethane
- Aluminum paints
- Epoxies
- Industrial enamel
- Urethane or polyurethane varnish

Special Areas To Consider

Attics

Allergic people should avoid attics because of the large amount of old dust that accumulates in them. If the attic space is finished with walls and painted, this exposure to old attic dust is eliminated. Frequently there are vents or open grills in the attic which draw air from the attic through the central heating system and into other areas of the home, thus creating exposure to attic dust. These should be sealed off, or designed out of new homes, so there is no air flowing between the attic and the interior of the home.

Basements and Split-Level Homes Below Ground

Cellars, basements, or rooms below ground are frequently cold and are sources of mold and dust. Unless they are moisture- and temperature-controlled or finished off, they should be eliminated from the design of the home. As with attics, care should be taken to assure that basement air does not mix with the air in the main part of the house, through cracks, air intakes for the heating system, or vents.

Entries

Allergenic sources, such as pollens, air pollutants, and molds come into the home through open doors and windows, as well as being carried in on clothing. To keep this air from the interior of the home, entrances should be made with enclosed foyers or separate rooms that can be closed off from the rest of the house. Coats and outerwear items can be stored in an adjacent closet within this area so that these items are never inside the living area of the home.

Garage

The location of an attached garage is important to the allergic person. For homes with an attached garage that do not have a breezeway between the garage and the home interior, a closed foyer entry is recommended. A garage beneath the home is potentially hazardous because it tends to fill with car fumes which seep into the home whenever the car is started. The same is true for any chemicals used in the garage. If the garage cannot be separated from the home, it should be well ventilated so that car and chemical fumes are dispersed outside. In addition, storage items should be kept in closed cabinets to eliminate this source of dust and molds. For homes in a design phase, a garage that is completely separate from the house is preferable.

Storage

Because of the restrictions for storage areas in the attic, basement, and garage, storage spaces may be limited. The chapter on allergy home control advises that only wash-and-wear items should be stored in a bedroom closet. Dry cleaned items, furs, and outdoor clothing need to be located in another part of the home. With all these considerations, storage space must be designed carefully into the home. Organized closet systems are ideal if they include closed cabinets as part of the design. Closets should be "walk-in" with enough space so that the clothes can be changed in the closet area. This prevents linters from spreading into the sleeping area.

Fireplaces and Bookshelves

Fireplaces are undesirable unless measures are taken to eliminate the sources for allergens. Glass screens can be used to keep pollens, drafts, and air pollutants out of the interior of the home. Glass or solid fronts for bookcases are also recommended because books are a potent source for dust and molds.

Kitchen

The kitchen has a number of potential sources that can cause physical symptoms. However, most of these are brought into the home and are not part of the construction. Basically, smooth finishes that can easily be cleaned should be considered for the cabinets, counters, floor, and walls. Electric stoves may be an advantage to some people because gas tends to be an irritant. The products from gas combustion combined with light contribute to interior air pollution. Exhaust ventilation should be installed to eliminate cooking odors and excessive moisture from cooking.

Bathrooms

Because moisture in a bathroom can be excessive, the materials selected for construction and decoration should resist moisture and be easy to clean. Tile can be a problem if not selected and installed carefully. The tiles should not be porous; in other words, the finish should be glazed. The grouting also should resist moisture so that water cannot get beneath tiles and cause mold or mildew to grow. Grout itself can support mold if not sealed with a silicone sealer. Glass doors on showers are preferable to plastic curtains because the doors clean easily. The glass door selected should be designed so that it does not require a track that harbors molds. Exhaust fans are needed to get rid of excessive moisture, and heating lights or a heater should be installed so that the room can be dried out. Storage areas should be covered with doors. All perfume or scented products should be kept in these areas.

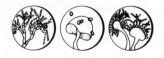

Interior Design Planning

Walls

Plaster or drywall should be the smoothest texture available. The rough texture varieties harbor vast amounts of dust and cannot be cleaned easily. Coving at the floor and ceiling also makes cleaning easier. (Materials used to decorate walls are covered more extensively in the chapter on decorating.)

Ceilings

Plaster or drywall with smooth texture, or smooth, synthetic acoustical ceilings are better than any ornate, decorative plasters. Even when they are textured, acoustical tiles made from synthetics are better to use than those made from animal or plant materials.

Flooring

The ideal floor consists of a smooth surface without cracks or seams. It should be made from nonporous materials that can withstand repeated, damp cleaning and should not be a source of dust itself. Asphalt tile, for example, will produce a fine dust if it has not been coated with acrylic.

Vacuum Systems

The ideal way to control dust in the home is through a central vacuum system. Standard cleaners expel fine particle dust back into the air, and they stay in the interior air of the home for a long time. A vacuum that takes the dust to an area where it can be exhausted outside is ideal.

The central vacuum system does not exhaust air back into the home. The vacuum system is installed in the garage, and pipes are installed while the home is being framed. Outlets for the system are located in various locations within the home. Only the hose and wand need to be connected to these outlets.

Homes already constructed can still have a central vacuum system, if the home has attic space, space beneath the home, or space between the floors. A contractor or installer can determine how the pipes can be most effectively placed.

Climate Control

Climate control in the home can be very complex, involving temperature, drafts, humidity, and interior air pollutants. A well-constructed home and a quality heating system are most desirable. However, not many homes, especially in the warmer climates, are built with allergic people in mind. Forced-air heating and air conditioning systems require special filters (see the following section on air filtration). In designing one of these systems, careful attention must be paid to air flows into and out of the system.

For purposes of understanding, the term "air conditioning" is used to refer to all aspects of air in the home: air cleaning, air cooling, heating, and humidification. The term "refrigeration" is used to refer to air which is conditioned to cool the home.

Evaporative cooling is not covered here. This type of cooling is not recommended for the allergic person because of the excessive moisture and mold problems that result from use of these units. By maintaining an even climate throughout the home, allergic symptoms can be better controlled.

Ideally, the home temperature should be maintained above 65 degrees Fahrenheit at all times and never over 75 degrees. In areas of the country where the temperature shifts quite a bit between night and day, some people have increased symptoms. Therefore 24-hour climate control is recommended. On the other hand, some people are aggravated by going from a cool refrigerated building to a hot exterior. Setting the refrigeration at a higher temperature so the shift is not as great makes these individuals feel better.

Controlling Air Quality

In order to control exterior air pollutants and allergens, the home should, ideally, be closed to the outside air at all times; however, this is not realistic because building codes frequently require mixing interior air with outside air. In addition, as we have already discussed, interior air pollutants actually build up in a closed environment. Depending upon individual needs, there are several ways to control this problem. Even if the air is filtered, sources for dust, molds or interior pollutants may still exist in the home or office. Filters can only filter moving air.

There are three ways to control indoor air pollution. One is to control the source of the exposure by elimination or substitution, the second is to dilute the air and the third is to remove it through filtration.

We control the sources for the dust, mold and air pollutants discussed earlier by eliminating them, or their byproducts, from the interior environment. It may be possible that a filter or exhaust at the source can eliminate the problem. The typical gas water heater, which has a vent so the combusted gases go up and out of the home, is an example of this method of controlling sources of pollution. Substituting different building or decorating materials is another way to eliminate the source of a potential pollutant. For example, 100 percent wood panel could be substituted for panels made with glues.

Dilution is a second way to control indoor air pollution. It can be accomplished in several ways. Air from outside can be brought into the home through natural ventilation; mechanical ventilation fans can be used; or the air within the home can be constantly circulated. Moving air around inside the home tends to dilute it.

The third way to control indoor pollutants is by moving the air out of the home by using an exhaust fan or by circulating it through a system of filters, either within one room or throughout the entire home.

THREE METHODS
FOR
CONTROLLING AIR POLLUTANTS

1• Control the source by removal, substitution or treatment.

2• Ventilate and dilute.

3• Filter or exhaust.

The circulation of air is very important when determining how to control the quality of air in a room, office or an entire building. If the construction professional is going to install a forced air system, the location of ducts that supply air and vents that return it to the system's filters is critical. The location of windows, doors, vented and unvented space heaters, and window or all refrigeration units must also be figured into the air flows. Ideally air should circulate from ceiling to floor throughout the whole room. For example, an office with cubicles will not have complete air circulation unless the cubicles are raised four inches off the floor.

Air Filtration

Ideally, the home should remain closed at all times to the outside air. If the interior design of the home is done carefully to avoid materials that produce dust or contain fibers and there are no chemical or off-gassing exposures, sophisticated airfiltration systems are not necessary. However, if a home has a forced-air heating system, a central filtration unit is recommended because the forced air keeps air particles from settling out of the air.

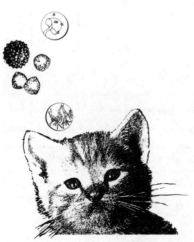

Particle Sizes

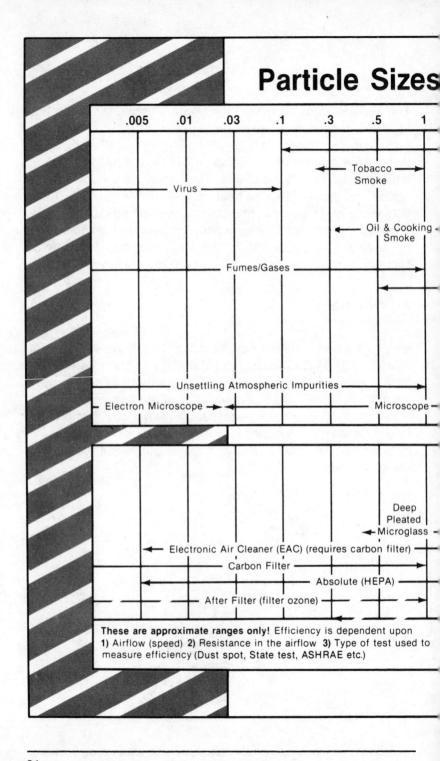

	.005	.01	.03	.1	.3	.5	1

Tobacco Smoke

Virus

Oil & Cooking Smoke

Fumes/Gases

Unsettling Atmospheric Impurities

Electron Microscope ←→ Microscope

Deep Pleated ← Microglass

← Electronic Air Cleaner (EAC) (requires carbon filter) →

Carbon Filter

Absolute (HEPA)

After Filter (filter ozone)

These are approximate ranges only! Efficiency is dependent upon
1) Airflow (speed) **2)** Resistance in the airflow **3)** Type of test used to measure efficiency (Dust spot, State test, ASHRAE etc.)

ilter Capabilities (in microns)

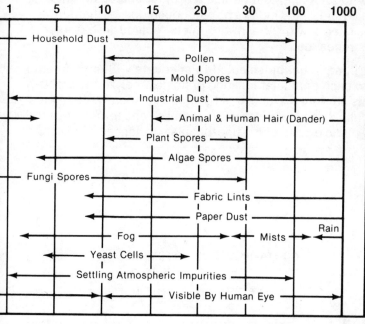

1	5	10	15	20	30	100	1000

Household Dust

Pollen

Mold Spores

Industrial Dust

Animal & Human Hair (Dander)

Plant Spores

Algae Spores

Fungi Spores

Fabric Lints

Paper Dust

Fog — Mists — Rain

Yeast Cells

Settling Atmospheric Impurities

Visible By Human Eye

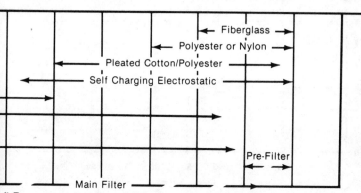

Fiberglass

Polyester or Nylon

Pleated Cotton/Polyester

Self Charging Electrostatic

Pre-Filter

Main Filter

4) Temperature/humidity **5)** Rigidity of frame **6)** Number of surfaces in the filter **7)** Cleanliness of filter (EAC inefficient if dirty, HEPA more efficient if dirty) The ideal filter has three stages (filters).

1 Micron = 1/25,000 inch.
For comparison, this period (.) is 200 micron in size.

Several factors are involved in adequate filtering. The first is the introduction of clean air, or ventilation. Fresh air may not be free of pollen or molds; therefore, outdoor air should enter the system just prior to filtering. Most homes rely on unfiltered air entering from the outside via windows or other openings, or through ventilation systems with "fresh air" inlets located in basements, attics, garages, etc.

Second, filters must be selected to adequately filter pollutants unique to each particular building or home. Analyze the problem pollutants in your particular situation. Are there particulates, house dust, chemicals, odors? It is important to consider the range of particle sizes of the undesirable substances. In the chart

CONTAMINANT VS EFFICIENCY

μ/cu.ft. = micrograms per cubic foot

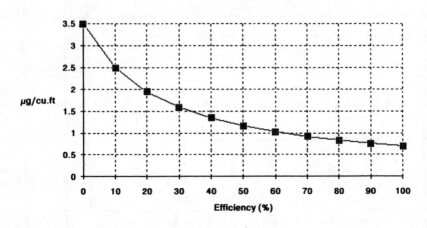

The graphs use the above relationship to show the sensitivity of indoor contamination to filter efficiency and to the contaminant concentration to filter air flow rate. In these examples, the following values were used:

Particle Sizes — Filter Capabilities, you can see that most pollens and bacteria are relatively large and easy to collect. In comparison, viruses and some fumes and gases that measure well into the sub-micron range require special filters.

Units that will filter one micron will meet the needs of most households. For people sensitive to house dust a filter with more capability is required.

Finally, consider the interrelationship of four factors: the efficiency of the filter, the flow rate of the air — that is, the number of times per hour the air is exchanged within a particular system — the amount of ventilation in the area, and the size of the area to be filtered.

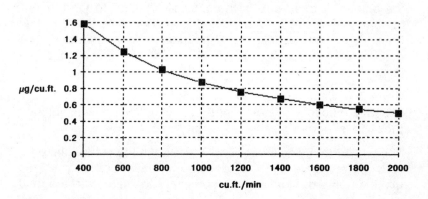

CONTAMINANT VS FLOW RATE

μ/cu.ft. = micrograms per cubic foot

Outside air contaminant level 2 micrograms per cubic foot.
Outside air ventilation rate 200 cubic feet per minute.
Indoor contaminant generation rate 300 micrograms per minute.

If one assumes that the amount of contaminants formed in the space plus that entering from the outside is equal to the amount filtered out and the amount displaced by the incoming air, the level of contaminants in the indoor air space will be approximately equal to the sum of the indoor particle generation rate and the rate of incoming contaminants in the outside air, that quantity divided by the sum of the outside air vent flow rate and the filter efficiency times the air flow through the filter. The following expression may be more clear:

$$\text{Contaminants} = \frac{\text{Inside Generation Rate} + \text{Outside Contaminant} \times \text{Ventilation Rate}}{\text{Ventilation Rate} + \text{Filter Efficiency} \times \text{Filter Flow Rate}}$$

EXAMPLE:

$$\text{Contaminants} = \frac{300 \ \mu\text{g/min} + 2 \ \mu\text{g/cu.ft} \times 200 \ \text{cu.ft./min.}}{200 \ \text{cu ft./min.} + .75 \ (\text{eff}) \times 600 \ \text{cu.ft/min.}}$$

$$= 0.875 \ \mu\text{g /cu.ft.} \quad \text{(or 3 } \mu\text{g/cubic meter)}$$

In reality we cannot assume that the amount of contaminants formed in the space plus that entering from outside is equal to the amount filtered out. In the case of off-gassing the amount of contaminants formed in the space will not all be filtered. Over time, there will actually be a build-up of contaminants. The number of times per hour of air exchanged will need to be increased.

If a high flow rate is required to ensure filtering, drafts in the room become noticeable. The air conditioning engineering will balance these four factors so this does not happen.

There is currently no recognized standard in the marketplace for rating filter efficiency in relationship to these four factors. This makes it very difficult for the consumer to evaluate the actual worth of the product or to evaluate conflicting information. The most useful test for comparing various products is the ASHRAE Dust Spot Test.

The ASHRAE Dust Spot Test is useful for comparing low efficiency filters. Since large particles account for most of the weight of the test dust, this test will not indicate how effective a filter is in removing the smaller particles in the 0.1 to 3.0 micron range.

The behavior of the various types of filters as they become loaded with dirt must be considered. In general, complex filters such as the HEPA (to be discussed next) that accomplish their filtration with purely mechanical means have a significant increase in their filtering capabilities as they load with dirt, since openings where particles pass through become smaller and smaller. Thus many manufacturers seek to rate the efficiency of their products at an average condition over the life of the filter.

This characteristic is true also for simple mechanical filters in a forced air system; however, since they have only light-duty air blowers, as they load with dirt, their air flow can drop and they actually become less efficient; the benefits from dirt load are not realized. The HEPA type filter becomes more efficient; its installation provides for pressure drop for a much longer period of time and it remains able to filter the smaller particle range.

The filter therefore needs to match the system into which it will be placed. The way to determine this is to find the rated air flow of the unit from the blower manufacturer. Then using the figure for the clean filter pressure drop available from the filter manufacturer, it can be determined whether or not the filter is suitable for the blower and how much pressure drop increase can be tolerated before the filter requires change. Your contractor or installer can readily answer this question for you.

In contrast to mechanical filters are particle filters that use electrostatic charge to assist in collection of fine particulate. There are two types; those with naturally charged fibers and electronic air cleaners. These filters most frequently show a decrease in capability as dirt accumulates, since dirt interferes with the electrostatic field. Thus frequent changing of the charged fiber filters and frequent cleaning of the electrostatic filters are beneficial. Electrostatic enhancement is most important for filtering submicron size particles.

Simple Filters

Fiberglass Filters

Many homes with forced-air heating include the inexpensive disposable fiberglass filters. These filters are not advised for anyone suffering from allergy or respiratory problems because they are inefficient.

Polyester Resinous Filter Media

Polyester resinous filter media comes by the roll and is disposable and fairly inexpensive. It can be cut to fit behind air registers and can be used as a filter for central forced-air heating. This type of media filters nearly 50 percent of the larger dust particles that pass through the media. Polyester filter media attracts dust by static force. It is quite effective for a mechanical filter. Some of this media is constructed with holes of graduated sizes that trap different sized particles.

Pleated Cotton Filter

In these filters, pleats increase filtering area capacity. They are disposable and usually made of non-woven reinforced cotton and synthetic filter media.

Polyurethane Foam

Permanent washable foam is quite inexpensive. It is used most frequently in the portable and window refrigeration units. This filter catches only large visible particles in the air. Foam can be cut to fit or bought in a frame.

Nylon Electrostatic Filter

The outer layers of woven nylon are stitched to an inner layer of open-cell polyurethane. It is really two different filters in one. It attracts particles by static force and traps only visible air particles.

Electrostatic Self-Charging Filter

An electrostatic self-charging filter is usually honeycombed or shredded plastic. The shredding increases the number of surfaces for the air to rub across, which sets up a static charge that attracts dirt particles. This is a permanent and inexpensive filter that is only efficient for filtering visible air particles.

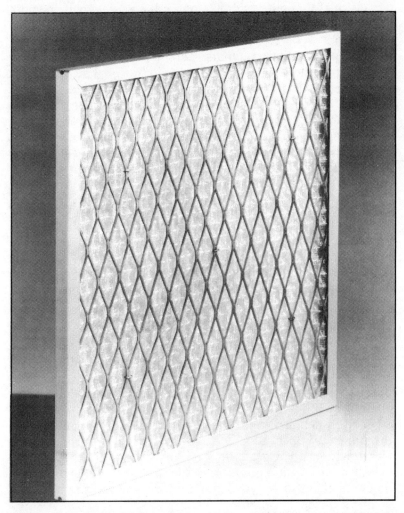

This **HI-TECH electrostatic filter can be vacuumed and reused for years. The frame with this permanent filter media can be made to fit your forced heating system. This filter serves as an excellent prefilter for a HEPA or Electronic Air Cleaner.**

Complex Filters

The filters already discussed do not filter out the very fine particles that can stay suspended in the air for long periods of time. However, they are useful in reducing the large particles around the environment and should be used in any home or office.

House dust that causes problems for the allergic person is not necessarily the dirt from outside that is blown into the home or is carried in on clothing. Dust is produced by the breakdown of plant and animal materials. Carpet pile, mattresses, pillow filling, attics, storage areas, and bookshelves are sources of this type of dust. The particle size of house dust is less than 5 microns, invisible to the eye. Linters from bedding, curtains, drapes, and clothing, for example, are up to l0 microns in size. Over time, however, these larger particles decompose to even smaller particles. Fungus or mold spores, bacteria, pollens and these larger dust particles can be filtered out of the air with electronic or absolute air cleaners.

Electronic air cleaners and absolute filters clean the flowing air very effectively. However, linting and dust sources will still exist. In some cases, the linting sources are so great that the electronic air cleaner cannot adequately filter the air. For this reason, it is necessary to remove heavy linters such as drapes, carpeting and bedspreads that are made from animal or plant fibers.

Electronic Air Cleaners

Two-stage electronic air cleaners are complex units that have a mechanical filter to catch large particles of dirt as the air first enters the cleaner. After this mechanical filter, the dirt-laden air passes to the first-stage or ionizing section, which negatively charges all dirt particles. The charged particles are collected on a positively charged metal plate that acts like a magnet to attract the particles. Up to 95 percent of airborne dirt is filtered and 99 percent of pollens are removed by this unit, if it is properly installed and maintained. The clean air is then passed through an optional activated-charcoal filter that removes air pollutants, such as gases or odors.

Electronic air cleaners can be installed in forced-air heating systems or can be purchased as individual units to place in a room. The portable electronic air cleaners are not as expensive as centrally installed units. Most of these units can service a closed area of about l5 by 20 feet. A unit can recirculate the air of a room this size four times each hour. If the room has an unusually high ceiling, or if the door is left open, the effectiveness of the filter is greatly reduced. This unit is designed for bedrooms, motel rooms, or other small areas. Many allergic people sensitive to pollen, mold, or dust have been helped by using one of these units at night.

Console electronic air cleaners, also portable units, are a little more expensive than the portable units and are much larger. They have a greater capacity and usually have two speeds for moving air.

In planning a home, the supplemental portable units may be all that is desired and may be the only alternative if perimeter or zone heating is used. If a forced-air heating system is used, the installation of a total system is recommended. A total system includes humidifier/dehumidifer, refrigeration, heating and electronic air cleaning. This will provide the maximum control of the interior climate of the home in addition to clean air.

Installation of a total system requires the design to be developd by an air conditioning engineer. This professional will figure the appropriate air flows, duct sizes, and equipment sizes required. This is very important for optimum functioning and climate control.

GUIDELINES FOR
ELECTRONIC AIR CLEANERS

1• Define your needs prior to shopping. Have you eliminated major dust sources? Have you figured the size of room(s) to be filtered? If you are installing a central forced air unit — are the ducts the appropriate size? Is there adequate air flow? Avoid a sales installation without analysis by an air conditioning engineer.

2• Follow cleaning schedule and manufacturer's instructions.

3• Change the pre-filter frequently to capture large particles to protect the electronic air cleaner.

4• Frequent arcing is not desirable. Clean and check the unit for broken wires, unusually large particles, moisture or anything unusual. Arcing produces ozone.

5• To avoid flash fire the carbon afterfilter should not be in contact with the electronic air cleaner.

Absolute Filters (HEPA)

The absolute filter, also called HEPA, a short term for high efficiency particulate air filter, is a multi-surfaced mechanical filter. The air is cleaned mechanically as it passes through the filter. No part of this filter is electrically charged. As this filter continues to operate, it becomes progressively more efficient because there are fewer pores for the particles to pass through. This type of filter does not produce any ozone. Eventually, the filter will have to be replaced, unlike the electronic air cleaner, which can be easily washed. The replacement is approximately 20 percent of the cost of the unit, and it will need to be replaced every year or two. HEPA filters require special engineering if they are installed in a central forced-air heating system. They are the most efficient filters available. HEPA filters are also available as portable units.

Use of Complex Filters

Both the electronic air cleaner and the HEPA filter should have what is called a prefilter, a mechanical filter such as a polyester filter, to remove large particles from the air. Another filter, called an afterfilter, can be installed behind the main filter. This filter is carbon, and it screens out air pollution, ozone, cigarette smoke, and cooking odors.

The electronic air cleaner and the HEPA filters should run 24 hours a day; otherwise, efficiency cannot be maintained. Windows should remain closed at all times to prevent outdoor pollutants from entering the home. If the proper furnishing is used in the home, the windows are kept closed, and the basic recommendations given in this book are followed, the home should be very clean.

At the end of this chapter a list of filter terms is provided for further clarification.

The Heating System

No matter what heating system is selected, proper equipment sizing is important. Do not select a heating installation company that uses "rule of thumb" figures if you expect an efficient system. Oversizing, as well as undersizing, of equipment can make true comfort an impossible dream.

The choice between the different recommended heating systems for the allergic person will depend on personal preference; cost and availability of gas, oil, or electricity; and the advice of a local qualified heating installer or air conditioning engineer.

Ideally, heat outlets will be under windows and at selected locations along the outer perimeter walls. This combination will help mix warm air with cold air at the source and prevent cold drafts. The proper number of cold air returns in a forced-air system is important to avoid cold areas and to provide efficient operation of an electronic air cleaner.

A large home, extensive glass areas, basements, and split levels all require special considerations that must be incorporated into the design of the heating system. The following describes some of the systems to consider.

Forced-Air Heating System

Forced-air heating systems are the biggest single source of allergic symptoms for persons who are sensitive to dust. Enormous amounts of dust are collected and circulated through these systems. Electronic air cleaners are recommended to remedy this situation. Forced-air heating systems, if properly sized and installed, can provide relatively comfortable heat for the home.

Electric Radiant Heat Panels

Electric radiant heat comes in a variety of systems, from a heated coil to panels that become part of the interior decor. One advantage of these units is that they can be located where heat is needed most. They are versatile because each room has its own heat source and does not depend on elaborate ducting throughout the home.

Radiant panels require electricity, which may not be practical in all locations. However, it is the cleanest form of heat available. There are no blowing fans or disturbing noises, and maintenance is convenient. Thermostatic control in each room provides zone control throughout a home.

Fan-Forced Electric Heaters

Small electric heaters can be installed flush to a wall or can stand free in a room. These units are recommended for auxiliary heating or for warm climates where heating is not a significant issue.

Electric Baseboard/Perimeter Heat/Hot-Water Heat

Strategically located electric or sealed hot-water heating systems can be located around the room on outside walls. Thermostats are located in each room to keep temperature even. This type of heating has several advantages over other types.

Humidification

As previously mentioned, humidity should be maintained between 40 to 60 percent. Many heating systems dry out the home during cold weather, and humidity may drop to as low as 10 to 15 percent. If some means of raising the humidity is not available, symptoms such as itchy skin or dry irritated respiratory passages will soon become apparent. For the sensitive allergic person, this can be quite an irritant. When humidity is below 30 percent, static electricity may cause irritating shocks, and room dust may increase because it does not settle as easily. A person may feel colder because of excess evaporation of moisture from the body. If the humidity is higher than 60 percent, molds grow more easily around the home, a situation that can also cause allergy symptoms.

If a home needs more humidity, an inexpensive method for adding moisture is the teapot or vaporizer. An hygrometer, an instrument for monitoring humidity, can be purchased. Some heating systems, such as water or steam heaters, have units added onto them for humidifying the air.

Power humidifiers are more accurate for the control of home humidity, especially for forced-air heating systems. These systems quickly adjust the humidity so that moisture shifts are not noticed. Portable units that can be moved around the home are available.

Dehumidification can be accomplished by portable units or central units installed in forced-air heating systems. This may be required if the home is damp during the winter. Forced-air, conditioning systems that include refrigeration automatically dehumidify as part of the cooling process.

Refrigeration

In many areas of the nation, refrigeration is necessary to keep the home within comfortable temperature limits. For efficient refrigeration, the home construction is as important as it is for heating the home. Insulation, weatherstripping and proper glass control are all vital to cooling a home.

The ducting requirements for centrally located refrigeration are the same as for electronic air cleaning. Therefore, a "total" system can be selected. If the home has baseboard electric or water heaters, wall or window air refrigeration units can be used.

Several refrigeration units have come onto the market over the years that include electronic air cleaning capability. The refrigeration section can be shut off, and the electronic air cleaner can still be used.

Refrigeration will be necessary if the home temperature cannot be maintained without heat buildup. Oversized refrigeration equipment may make occupants feel clammy because it cools down the house quickly, then goes off. While it is off, the humidity quickly climbs. However, the temperature rises more slowly, and the thermostat does not trigger the system until it is a certain temperature. As with all of this equipment, proper installation is very important.

Odor Control

For the allergic person, odors can be irritating and possibly a source for symptoms. Attempting to cover up odors in a home also may be a source for symptoms. Therefore, special attention must be given to methods of control.

Masking

Masking odor is accomplished in two ways: by desensitizing the ability to detect odors and by introducing a stronger or more acceptable odor to cover the undesirable one.

Nasal desensitization occurs when ozone is injected into the atmosphere from a mechanical device. A high discharge of electrical energy reduces the sensitivity of the tender membranes in the nose. High concentrations of ozone will break down these odors; however, ozone in the air can be harmful. Ozone in non-toxic amounts will not eliminate odors, although it will reduce the ability to perceive them. This method of masking odor is best avoided by anyone who is allergic.

Artificial odors are available to cover existing odors. They do not remove the odors or control them and in themselves may be a source for allergy symptoms.

Combustion

Although fire is one of the oldest known methods of destroying odors, it is not effective unless complete combustion takes place. Incomplete combustion is undoubtedly the greatest contributor of smog and air pollutants today.

Ventilation

The intake, circulation, and removal of air has been widely accepted as a method to control odors. However, depending on the air source, the allergic person may be affected by the allergens in the incoming air. Circulation of "inside" air is acceptable for the allergic person.

Removal

Another means of controlling odors is removal by power exhaust and by sorption, whereby the odor molecules are taken out of the air by special filters. Activated carbon, liquid scrubbers, and other special absorbing and adsorbing filters can be used.

High heat and humidity can adversely affect the functioning of activated charcoal, eventually causing previously collected odors to be discharged back into the air stream. The critical factor is the carbon's true capability to retain odors, since it does not actually destroy them. If a home has carbon filters, they should be changed at the recommended intervals to avoid these problems.

FILTER TERMS

We have listed a few key filter terms below as a reference. Although a filter expert modified some of these definitions, the original source is unknown.

ABSORBERS • Filters that take up gases and engulf them to several times their weight.

ADSORBERS • Filters that collect gases in a condensed form on a surface.

AIR FILTER • A device utilized to remove airborne contaminants.

AIR PURIFIERS • Small forced air devices that may utilize charcoal, silica gel and other filters, sometimes a HEPA filter. They filter very small areas.

ANOMETER & VELOMETER • Instruments which measure the velocity of the air.

APPROACH VELOCITY • The velocity of the air as it approaches an air handling device (the filter area).

APPARATUS HOUSE • The box-like structure that houses the fan, coils, filter bank, fresh air dampers and return air dampers. The chambers at each end are referred to as the PLENUM.

ARRESTANCE — (ASHRAE) • Gravimetric efficiency on ASHRAE test dust.

ASHRAE 52-76 • Test method for air filters covering efficiency, arrestance, and dust loading.

ATMOSPHERIC DUST • The term atmospheric dust is used to designate the particulate matter naturally occurring in the air supplied to the test duct.

BYPASS • This refers to unfiltered air going around the filter because it has not been properly sealed in place.

CAPACITY • The volume of air (CFM) which can be delivered through a filter unit.

RATED CAPACITY • That CFM rating which is specified by the manufacturer.

CFM (CUBIC FEET PER MINUTE) • A measure of the volume of air being used in a system. An air handling system rated at 20,000 CFM would have a volume of air equal to 20,000 cubic feet entering the plenum every minute. CFM = FPM x flow cross-sectional area.

CONTAMINANTS • Airborne dirt, dust spores, viruses, bacteria and allergens which are sometimes referred to as AEROSOLS.

DEPTH LOADING • A characteristic of fiber media. Measured as the ability of the media to distribute dirt through its total depth, as opposed to surface or face loading. Typically, pure lint will face load a filter.

DOWNSTREAM • The air exit side of a filter or such equipment or areas located after a filter system.

D.O.P. • Dioctyl phthalate; a test aerosol used for absolute filters in accordance with military standards.

DUST HOLDING CAPACITY • The gram weight of dust, or contaminants, that is captured by a filter before the resistance rises to a specified level at a specified velocity. It equals the dust fed times the average arrestance.

EFFICIENCY • Effectiveness on removal of atmospheric dust using the discoloration or "dust spot" method.

ELECTRONIC AIR CLEANER • These devices clean air by flowing air past an electrode that gives airborne particles a relatively strong electrical charge. The air then passes collector plates having the opposite electrical charge to which the particles adhere.

FACE LOADING • The phenomenon by which certain contaminants in the air load up on the surface of the filter media. Filter life is usually shortened when this occurs.

FIBER BREAK OFF • Particles of the media fiber breaking off and entering the airstream. Under normal circumstances this is inconsequential.

FPM (FEET PER MINUTE) • The speed (velocity) of the air at a given point in the air handling system. FPM = CFM − area.

FRESH AIR • Outdoor air that is free from local pollution sources.

HEPA • High Efficiency Particulate Air (HEPA) filters, originally developed for military use. Efficiencies range from 95-99.99% D.O.P.

HIGH EFFICIENCY • Normally considered 50-95% average dust spot efficiency. (ASHRAE 52-81).

LOFT • Thickness of filter media, generally used to describe how fibers are distributed.

LOW EFFICIENCY • Efficiencies under the 20% range on atmospheric dust. Low efficiency examples: Fiberglass media, fiberglass disposables, standard polyester, roll filters.

MAXIMUM ALLOWABLE RESISTANCE • Recommended final pressure drop by manufacturer at rated air flow.

MEDIA • Plural of medium. Materials in a filter which filter the air.

MEDIA MIGRATION • Carry-over of fibers from a filter into the discharge air. Similar to fiber break-off.

MEDIA VELOCITY • Average rate of speed of the air through a filter. It is defined as the air flow rate divided by the net effective filtering area. This term has no meaning for electronic devices which collect dust on permanent electrodes.

MICRON OR MICROMETER • A unit of length in the metric system. One millionth of a meter, 10^{-4} centimeter, 10^{-3} millimeter, or 0.00039 of one inch.

DIRT MIGRATION • The process by which dirt releases itself from the media fibers and enters the airstream and becomes a contaminant.

OFF-GASSING • Gasses given off into the air as the drying or aging process takes place in a new building or whenever new decorative materials have been installed in a room.

NONSUPPORTED MEDIA • Filters in which the pleats are extended and supported in the air stream only by the airflow, with no separate media support.

PREFILTER • Filter utilized to reduce dirt loading to subsequent filters (usually higher in efficiency).

PRESSURE DIFFERENTIAL • The difference in static pressure between the upstream and downstream side of the filter.

RESISTANCE • Resistance is the loss of static pressure caused by the filter, usually expressed in inches, measured to the nearest 1.01 in. Velocity=CFM ÷ area.

RETURN AIR • Air which has been returned from occupied spaces in a building for recirculation. Return air will generally be introduced and mixed with incoming fresh air before filtration.

SUPPORTED MEDIA • Filters in which the filtration media is supported by wires, separators, etc. It is usually in pleated form.

U L Ratings - CLASS 1 & 2 • Flammability and smoke ratings applied to filters by J. Allergy Clin. Immunol 64:3-4, 1979.

UNLOADING • The process by which dirt, originally stopped by the filter, is released back into the airstream.

UPSTREAM • The air entering the side of the filter.

VELOCITY • Rate of the speed of the air through a filter. It is defined as the air flow rate divided by the net effective filtering area. This term has no meaning for electronic devices which collect dust on permanent electrodes.

7
ALLERGY HOME CONTROL

Maintaining an allergen-free environment will enhance the factors an allergic person needs to keep in balance or control. More than one-third of the day is spent in the home, so it is most important to control or eliminate allergens in this location.

First of all, the home must be easy to keep clean. Converting a home to an allergy-free environment can be expensive, and it may be wise to eliminate items gradually as they wear out, replacing them with furnishings made of allergy-free materials. Drapes, rugs, bedding, and so on that contain animal and plant materials should be avoided. Synthetic materials, which resist dust and molds, should be used instead.

Chapter Three covered molds and environmentals, including dust and other plant and animal fibers, that can cause symptoms of allergy. Once you know the sources for these allergens, the next step is to find ways to eliminate them from the environment.

GUIDELINES FOR
MOLD AVOIDANCE

✦ Keep air circulating in the home. Avoid closing up the home for more than a day or two without any circulation of air.

✦ Keep new shower curtains free from mildew, and soak them in saltwater before hanging them. (If the curtain is mildewed, spread baking soda on it and wipe it clean.)

✦ Do not put damp clothes in a hamper.

✦ Iron dampened clothes immediately.

✦ Use water-and-mildew-resistant sealers around tubs and sinks, on cement floors, and on underground walls.

✦ Use exhaust fans in bathrooms and kitchen.

✦ Leave a light on in damp bathrooms or closets.

✦ Vent dryers to the outdoors.

✦ Use a dehumidifier if humidity is higher than 60 percent.

✦ Avoid use of evaporative coolers in the home.

✦ Wash walls and floors with solutions that continue to inhibit mold growth after the solutions dry. Examples include Zepherin or you can mix three tablespoons trisodium phosphate in one-half cups bleach in one gallon of water.

✦ Store books, magazines, and newspapers behind sealed doors or storage areas. The storage area should not be in or near the bedroom.

✦ Rid the home of cardboard boxes and storage items that are not packed and sealed.

✦ If the home is damp, heat it until it dries.

— CONTINUED —

> ✦ Use mold-inhibiting paints in damp areas of the home.
>
> ✦ If molds continue to be a problem, request a fungal survey to identify the type of mold and to quantify the extent of the exposure. Your physician can then use skin tests to see if you are allergic to the mold.

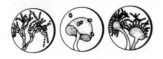

ELIMINATING DUST, MOLDS AND ENVIRONMENTALS

Some practical guidelines are recommended to make it easy to keep a home clean.

Carpet and Floors

If carpeting is used in the home, it should not contain animal or plant fiber, such as cotton or wool. Carpeting should be 100 percent synthetic fibers. The sculptured patterns, high-low patterns, or short shags are well suited for allergy control. Twisted pile and looped pile are not desirable because they harbor dust more easily. The carpet pad must be of a synthetic material or rubber.

Carpeting should be dry-cleaned or steam-cleaned every year. Although dry cleaning with chemicals is ideal, the cleaning process may affect an allergic person. It is best to stay away while the carpet is being cleaned, possibly for a day or two afterward. Carpet shampoos are not recommended because they leave residue particles in the fibers that when disturbed, float into the air.

To keep carpeting as dust-free as possible, use a vacuum cleaner that has strong suction. Especially desirable are the internal vacuum systems. A central vacuum is located in a garage or workroom, and a system of pipes runs to strategic parts of the home. A hose and wand are used to pick up the dirt, and it is transported to the central unit. This type of system does not exhaust fine dust back into the home's air.

Exhausted vacuum air is contaminated with very small dust particles, highly potent to the person who is allergic to dust. The allergic person should not vacuum unless such a system is used. Expensive vacuum systems are available that use filtration through water to make the exhaust clean; however, because of their cost, they are not recommended. Furthermore, the companies that manufacture most of these vacuum systems promote use of the system for humidification as well as for some other procedures. Because these other uses can put bacteria into the air, they are not recommended. As long as the allergic person is out of the home during vacuuming, a powerful vacuum can be used. The bags should be disposable and should be changed very frequently. The allergic person should not be in the home during vacuuming. Circulate air through the room or home for about fifteen minutes to eliminate fine particle dust in the air.

The ideal floor surface is one that has a hard nonporous surface and can be damp-mopped. Wood, tile, stone, and vinyls are ideal. Waxes and products used to shine the floor surface should be avoided. They will not be necessary if floors are sealed properly. Most vinyl floors require no sealing and no maintenance chemicals. Older floors such as asphalt, vinyl asbestos, or linoleum need to be sealed with acrylic sealer. Asphalt is porous and very dusty. As linoleum floors age, the black layer that becomes exposed is asbestos, a health hazard.

Walls and Ceilings

Wall and ceiling surfaces should be smooth and nonporous. For rough plaster or textured surfaces, a variety of sealers and paints can be used. Textured plaster can be painted with a semigloss latex-base paint; a masonary surface can be sealed; and wood surfaces can be sealed with clear coats. These sealers will keep dust from adhering to the surface and make it easy to wipe the surface clean.

Wall coverings are suitable if they are vinyl and can be washed. Synthetic water-base glues are recommended. Older glues were made with wheat paste, a great source for mildew when walls are damp.

Newer acoustical ceilings made of plastic gunite are safe. However, older homes frequently have acoustical ceilings made of asbestos or flax bound with animal glues. Both the flax and the glue are potential allergens. Some of these old ceilings can be painted with a vinyl-base paint that will not destroy the sound-absorbing quality of the ceiling, and it will decrease exposure to the allergens.

Furniture

The ideal furniture will have a hard, smooth surface. Examples are plastic, enameled wood, metal and fine wood with a clear-coat finish.

To clean fine furniture finishes, use a dust cloth treated with a silicone for static attraction. Avoid oiled woods and furniture cleaned with aerosol furniture cleaners or creams. Some of the oils used to condition woods cause allergic symptoms. Generally, the finer the oil is, the better. Read the label. Oils from cottonseed frequently cause problems.

Upholstered furniture is acceptable if the interior fill is a synthetic, such as polyester, and the exterior fabric is also synthetic. Avoid goose down, flax, and kapok fillers. When buying new furniture, inquire about all the materials used in the construction, not simply the fiber content of the upholstery fabric.

The best choices in upholstery fabric are synthetic fibers, such as polypropylene, olefin, nylon, orlon, rayon or any synthetic blend that is tightly woven. Leather is not recommended because it contains chemicals used in its treatment that can be irritants. If you have upholstery fabric that is made of natural fibers, it can be sprayed with dust retardants. Ask the fabric maker what is recommended. Commercially available dust retardants called Dust Seal and Allergex can be used. The retardant should be applied every six months. Soil repellents are not necessary; synthetic fibers naturally repel soil, but not serious spills.

The Bedroom

Because about one-third of the day is spent in the bedroom, it is most important to keep it as free from dust and mold as possible. If you can make your bedroom a haven from allergens and thus enhance your chances of getting a good night's sleep, you are more likely to keep physically balanced. It is obvious then that the bedroom is the number-one priority in your control of the environment.

Proper care and furnishing of the bedroom is much like that for the entire home; however, stricter measures are usually needed. Clutter, which collects dust, must be eliminated. Books, magazines, toys, and other objects kept in the bedroom should be put away in closed cabinets and drawers.

Stuffed toys should be washable and filled with polyester, nylon stockings, or particle foam. If a child is especially attached to a stuffed toy filled with allergenic material such as flax or kapok, that stuffing can be removed and replaced with one of the recommended fillers. Perfumes and cosmetic products, often kept on dresser tops, can cause allergy symptoms and should be kept elsewhere.

Because carpeting is a natural dust collector, the bedroom of an allergic person should not be carpeted. A smooth floor surface, such as vinyl, is ideal. Asphalt or wood flooring is suitable only if it is sealed with polyurethane or acrylic floor sealers. The Swedish floor finishes are suitable on fine wood floors because they can be damp-wiped. Other surface coatings such as wax can actually cause allergic reactions in some persons. Synthetic throw rugs that can be washed frequently are acceptable in the bedroom. If a carpet cannot be removed, the previously mentioned suggestions for suitable carpet care should be followed.

Special attention must be paid to the bed. Mattresses and box springs, even so-called hypoallergenic or nonallergenic mattresses, should be encased in nonporous, zippered encasings. This is necessary because the dust mite is harbored in the bedding. Many department stores carry a variety of these encasings, but the best ones are made especially for allergic persons and can be ordered from a catalog. (See the products index at the end of the book.) Less-expensive, four-gauge vinyl encasings are available, but they often have fused seams that tear apart easily. For comfort, two bottom sheets could be used over the encasings if the vinyl feels too warm. New encasings should be aired for a day or two because the new odor can be irritating.

Blankets should be made of synthetic fibers that can be washed frequently. Do not use wool or cotton blankets. Use of flannel sheets during the winter is suitable only if they are washed frequently when they are new to get rid of lint.

Bedspreads must be washable and should be laundered monthly. Quilted, washable bedspreads filled with polyester and made with synthetic fibers are attractive and safe. Polyester and cotton blends are good for allergy control. Do not use chenille or 100 percent cotton, wool, or other natural-fiber bedspreads.

Sheets should be washed weekly. Avoid 100 percent cotton and muslin sheets because they produce lint. The 60 percent polyester/cotton, 100 percent polyester, and nylon sheets are all recommended. Mattress pads also should be filled with polyester

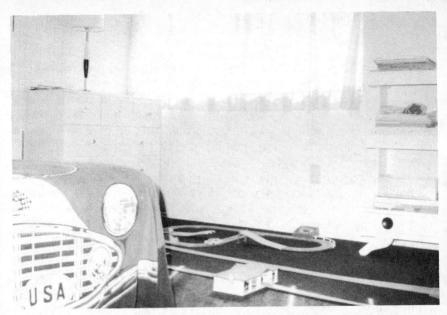

An Ideal Boy's Bedroom. A washable cotton/polyester bedspread and washable nylon curtains are the only items requiring extra attention. The carpet is ozite that takes cleaning and scrubbing. The furniture is enameled latex paint and the wallcovering is vinyl.

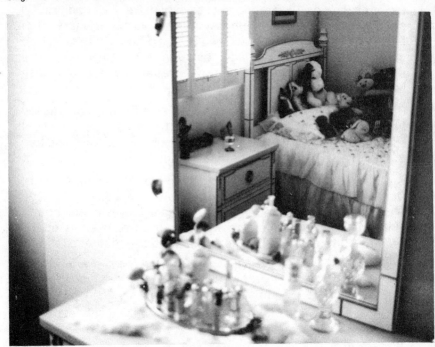

Young Girl's Bedroom that Was Ideal. This bedroom has all the appropriate decorative fibers to avoid dust making sources, i.e. enameled latex painted shutters, nylon bedspread, mattress and box springs encased with nonporous encasings and art prints covered with glass. However, the animals are filled with a mixture of kapok, flax and cotton filling and the perfume over the rabbit pelt are problems that should be removed from the room.

or synthetic fibers and should be washed each time the sheets are washed. If mites are present, this source will be eliminated.

Inexpensive polyester pillows should be placed in zippered encasings. Avoid the use of feather pillows even if they are encased. If there is a second bed in the room, it should be treated the same as the one the allergic person uses.

When washing bedding, follow the washing instructions to avoid the residue from fabric softeners, soaps, and conditioners.

Bedroom closets also should be kept allergen-free. Only washable clothing should be hung free in the closet. Keep dry-cleaned garments and storage items in zippered plastic bags. Interior closet surfaces should be smooth and painted, just as the walls and ceilings of the bedroom are. Cardboard boxes or clothing used for outdoor activities should be kept in a closet in another part of the home. Ideally, no cardboard should be present in the home. Do not store vacuum cleaners, cleaning products, or any hobby chemicals in the bedroom.

Do not use moth crystals in the bedroom closet. Moth killers are unnecessary if the closet is full of synthetic fibers because moths attack only animal and plant fibers. If the closet is damp, a light bulb left on will keep the closet dry and reduce mold growth.

If windows tend to drip moisture, measures should be taken to keep the area dry. Placing a towel at the window base each day may catch the moisture. The towel should be washed and dried each time it is used on the window. Double-paned windows or storm windows should solve the moisture problem.

Climate Control of the Home

The ideal interior climate in the home is between 65 and 72 degrees Fahrenheit. The humidity should be between 40 and 60 percent. If a refrigeration air conditioner is used, the temperature should be set no less than 12 degrees below the outside temperature.

Air Cleaning

The chapter on building covered the different kinds of filters that can be used in the home. This aspect of cleaning the home is very important, but not as important as eliminating dust-producing sources in the home.

CLEANING AND CLEANING PRODUCTS

The Laundry

Over a period of time, soaps, fabric softeners, starch, and fabric conditioners build up and make clothes dull and gray and stiff to the touch. These substances can be removed with the proper use of sodium combinations such as Calgon or laundry soda. If you have soft water or water-conditioning equipment, washing clothing once a month with one cup of Calgon or laundry soda will keep the laundry residue-free. If you do not have water-softening equipment or naturally soft water, use water-softening chemicals, especially during the rinse cycle.

With soft water, use biodegradable soap or detergent in very limited amounts, usually about one-half cup. With hard water, a low-suds detergent is usually the best choice. Avoid detergents with additives or conditioners. Sometimes the conditioners coat the fabric to leave it soft, and a residue remains. Do not use liquid fabric softeners. Fabric softener sheets can also be a problem because of their scent.

If you use an automatic clothes dryer, the exhaust should be vented to the outside to avoid lint dispersion in the garage or home. Line drying allows clothing to pick up allergens such as pollens, air pollutants, and molds.

Clothes hampers are frequently a source of molds because clothes may be damp. Empty hampers frequently, and disinfect the inside to kill mold spores. Do not shake laundry items inside the home or laundry area.

Disinfectants

Disinfectants are useful for control of the bacteria in clothing. Four types are available: quaternary, liquid chlorine, pine oil, and phenolic.

Quaternary disinfectants are colorless and odorless compounds that are effective at all temperatures. Benzalkonium chloride and/or n-alkyl benzyl ammonium chloride should be listed as an ingredient on the label. These products are the best choices.

Liquid chlorine disinfectants are relatively inexpensive, readily available, and effective at all temperatures. The label should state that the product contains 5.25 percent sodium hypochlorite.

Pine oil disinfectants are effective in hot and warm water. The label should state that the product contains orthobenzyl-parachlorophenol or orthophenyl-chlorophenol.

Cleaning Tips

Your cleaning arsenal should be limited to the basics such as soda, salt, vinegar, borax, and Calgon. All the aerosols, strong odorous chemicals, paste waxes, and solvent cleaners should be removed from the home.

The following bedroom cleaning cycles are recommended:

1• Thorough cleaning of the bedroom (walls, floor, and closet).

  ✓ Clean every four to six weeks if allergy symptoms occur.

  ✓ Clean every two to four months if the allergic person is symptom-free.

  ✓ Clean every six months if the room is filtered for particles below 5 microns.

2• Blankets and bedspreads

  ✓ Wash every four to six weeks if the allergic person is having symptoms.

3• Floors

  ✓ Vacuum carpeting twice a week.

  ✓ Damp-mop hard floors twice a week.

4• Furniture/shelves/woodwork

  ✓ Damp wipe weekly.

Rearranging and cleaning a storage room or garage may result in exposure to highly potent allergens; therefore, an allergic person doing the cleaning should wear a face mask. You can buy disposable paper masks or make your own from dense fabric. Remember, however, that only large particles will be filtered out by the mask. A person who is allergic really should not do this type of work.

Avoid sweeping or dusting with a dry cloth. Sweeping and dry dusting spreads dust thoroughly throughout the room. A damp dust cloth will ensure that dust is picked up and not dispersed into the air. A silicone-treated cloth is also suitable.

Chemical dust retardants marketed under the brand names Allergex and Dust Seal are available. These products can be used in areas where you cannot afford to replace a natural-fiber item with a synthetic one.

Waxing floors is not advisable. However, the acrylic liquids seem to cause fewer symptoms and dry faster than wax. Many fumes from wax products trigger allergic reactions, especially if the home has gas utilities.

A product that aids in cleaning is liquid fabric softener. Use full-strength fabric softener on surfaces that collect dust such as heater grills, Venetian blinds, lamp bases, or decorative grills or screens. Applying a diluted solution to walls after they are scrubbed will help repel dust. Acrylic coatings can be used on any porous surface to help repel dust. Adhesive papers such as Contact can be used inside drawers or closets to create a smooth, wipable surface.

If you have followed the decorating recommendations in this book, you have no drapes or curtains to take down and hang up for frequent cleaning. You can damp-wipe most items, further reducing exposure to dust. You will not have dust balls beneath the beds to clean because you have encased the mattress and box springs. You will not be able to write your name in the dust on tables within a few days.

To assist you in finding causes of allergy symptoms in your home, a check list has been provided as a guide for possible sources for allergens. Once they are identified, you can either eliminate the source or follow one of the recommendations made in the book.

ALLERGY ENVIRONMENT CHECKLIST

List environmental allergens to eliminate:

HOME AND LOCATION

Prevailing wind from _____

Name possible sources for problems in the prevailing wind: [traffic, industry, cultivated farm land (name crops), large body of water, marshlands, grove (name trees), golf course, fields or open space (see what common weeds are in the area);]

Home Site

_____ Rural

_____ City

_____ Adjacent fields

_____ Nearby ditches

_____ Bulldozing or large construction project in area

_____ Windy exposure

_____ Canyon site or nearby canyon

_____ Large area of repeated landscaping; i.e., bermuda grass, trees that line the streets, shrubs common to most of the homes in the area, planted parkways, etc.

_____ Nearby corrals, chicken pens, or other animals
_____ Other:

Home Construction and Maintenance

_____ Insecticides used around home foundation.
Name:

_____ Foundation of cement. If yes, is the slab sealed with plastic? If no, check cement for dampness.
_____ Basement. Are there cement walls next to soil? If yes, check for dampness.
_____ Is foundation above ground? If yes, is underside of home sealed, including vents?
_____ Is there an attic? If yes, are there any vents, pipes, or openings that communicate into the home?

Forced-Air Systems

_____ Is there forced-air heating? If yes, Are the cold air intakes drawing air from attic, underside of home, outdoor air, or basement?
_____ Is there forced-air refrigeration?
_____ Is there an electronic air cleaner? If yes, when was it last serviced and checked for efficiency?
_____ What type of mechanical filter is used in the system? How often is it cleaned or changed?

Cleaning Products used in the home

List all cleaning products used in the home.

Do the labels indicate possible allergens or irritants?
Are the products scented? Are they aerosol?

List all toiletries and cosmetics used in the home.
Do the labels indicate possible allergens or irritants?
Are the products scented? Are they aerosol?

Is the vacuum cleaner efficient? How often is the home vacuumed? How often is the collecting bag replaced?

Animals

_____ Cat, dog, furred pets or other (name)_____ in the home? All the time? (Yes) ☐   No) ☐

Allergy Sufferer's Bedroom:

_____ Is the fill in pillow(s) other than synthetic? Are the pillows encased?
_____ Is the mattress(s) encased with nonporous zippered encasing?
_____ Are the box springs encased?
_____ Are blankets a tight-weave synthetic fiber?
_____ Is bedspread made with a synthetic fiber and filled with a synthetic fiber? Is it washable?
_____ Are sheets a fine weave such as percale, at least 50 percent polyester, nylon, or satin?
_____ Are there any articles on the bed such as back rests, stuffed toys or animals? If so, are they filled with synthetic fibers?

Washing methods for bedding:

_____ Are blankets washed every 4-6 weeks?
_____ Is bedspread washed every 2 months?
_____ Are sheets washed weekly?
_____ Are sheets treated with a fabric softener?

_____ What brand of soap is used?

_____ Are additives used in the rinse cycle? If yes, is Calgon, or laundry soda used?

_____ Is soft water used to wash clothes? If no, is Calgon or laundry soda added to the wash cycle?

Furnishings:

List each piece of furniture in the room and indicate if it has any of the following:

_____ Is upholstery fabric synthetic?

_____ Is upholstery fill synthetic?

_____ Is furniture ornate or does it contain many holes or crevices to harbor dust? (as in rattan, for example)

_____ Is the finish of the furniture smooth and easily damp-wiped? If furniture is oiled, what product is used to oil it?

_____ What furniture creams or cleaners are required? Are they sources for allergy?

Other items in the bedroom

List other items in the room that may catch or make dust.

_____ Lamp shades

_____ Wall decor

_____ Decorator pillows

Windows

_____ Broken? If yes, repair.

_____ Air leaks? If yes, weatherstrip with synthetic material.

_____ Damp or decayed wood around window?

_____ Sweating of windows? If yes, how is the sill or floor kept dry?

_____ Are there mold stains around the window, wall, or floor?

_____ Does window remain closed all the time? If no, can filter be installed to filter incoming air?

ALLERGY ENVIRONMENT CHECKLIST *CONTINUED—*

Window Treatment

_____ Shades? Washable?

_____ Shutters? Smooth enamel finish?

_____ Drapes? Washable? Dry-cleaned? Drapes are not recommended. If they cannot be removed, can they be washed frequently?

_____ Curtains? Washable? Dry-cleaned? If they cannot be removed, can they be washed or cleaned frequently?

_____ Vertical blinds? How can they be cleaned?

_____ Mini blinds?

_____ Other type window covering? Can it be damp-cleaned easily?

Floor

_____ Tile? Is the grout sealed with silicone?

_____ Sheet flooring? If not vinyl or sealed with polyurethane, is the floor smooth and nonporous?

_____ Wood? Is the surface sealed?

_____ How is the floor cleaned? Are any strong chemicals used?

_____ Carpet? Is the pile and fiber suitable for good allergy control?

_____ Carpet pad? How old is the pad?

Personal Habits

_____ Does allergy sufferer take natural vitamins? (natural ingredients such as cod liver oil, herbs, etc.)

_____ Do the cleaning?

_____ Have a hobby or activity that exposes to chemicals?

_____ Mow the lawn? Near mowing?

_____ Work around office machines, chemicals, or in a dusty environment?

8
♦

DECORATING THE HOME

A DECORATING PHILOSOPHY

Yesterday the allergic person was required to live in a clinic-like atmosphere. Today, with a little ingenuity, the home can be decorated delightfully. The austere feeling has been eliminated by using materials recently developed through science.

Because allergies are constantly changing, a room furnished with completely synthetic materials is the most desirable. The conversions in decor that may be suggested are costly. You can hold expenses to a minimum.

Once you have followed the suggested methods for cleaning set forth in the last chapter, the home is bare and uninviting. When you are selecting fibers and materials for decorating, a few basic rules will help you avoid allergenic sources and, at the same time, simplify housecleaning. By carefully selecting decorative fibers that will not break down, the home will not be as dusty.

Basically, try to avoid having any animal or plant fibers in the home because these fibers decompose to make dust. The synthetic fibers can hold airborne dust but they do not break down to form allergenic dust. Avoid any fibers that will lint or that have a loose weave because loosely woven fibers catch and hold airborne dust. Dust catchers such as drapes, unwashable bedspreads, comforters, knick-knacks, or other ornate objects should be eliminated. Any fiber you select should be guaranteed washable, should not shed or pill, and should be woven with synthetic fibers. Any new synthetic fibers brought into the home should be washed or aired to rid the fabrics of irritable chemicals present when the fabrics are new.

SOUND-ABSORBING MATERIALS

Whenever you remove sound absorbers such as drapes, upholstered furniture, carpets, and built-in acoustical materials of animal and plant fibers, you may end up with an easy-to-clean home but a noisy one. There are several ways to remedy this situation.

A resilient floor absorbs considerable sound, and with any carpeting, the problem is lessened. Carpet padding will absorb sound, and it will help keep noise from traveling from floor to floor. Because of its sound-absorbing qualities, cushion vinyl flooring is wonderful in kitchens, family rooms, bathrooms, and even bedrooms. The new acoustical materials on the market can be washed easily. Some of the newer acoustical ceilings that are applied through a blowing process are made of plastics. Even if you have the older type of acoustical ceiling that is made with flax and animal glues, it can be painted to seal the allergenic sources without losing much sound-absorbing ability.

Upholstered furniture with the proper materials recommended for the allergic person will still have a good sound-absorbing ability.

FLOORING

An ideal floor has a nonporous texture and a smooth surface without cracks or seams. It should be able to take repeated damp cleaning and not be a source of dust.

Vinyl sheets are the best selection for bathrooms, kitchens, and other actively used rooms. The sheets should be 100 percent vinyl and should be installed with as little seaming as possible. Tile vinyl is satisfactory, but each crack becomes a source for dirt. Avoid textured patterns; they collect dirt and are not easily cleaned. Vinyl floors should be coved at the sides to prevent a dirt zone along the base of each wall.

Some other examples of desirable floors are terrazzo, marble, smooth stone such as slate, and sealed wood. Carpeting is suitable if specific requirements are followed. Carpet and carpet pads are discussed at the end of this section. If you wish to have wood floors, they should be finished with a sealer that allows for damp mopping. The newer seamless vinyl floors, which are actually poured on, are also ideal.

The following descriptions of different types of flooring include recommendations for the allergic person.

Asphalt Tile

Asphalt tile has a full thickness of asphaltic or resinous binder with asbestos or other fibers, fillers, and pigments. It is formed under pressure while hot. The finished product is porous and hard to keep clean because of its dust-making quality. It is not desirable for the allergic person unless it is sealed with a heavy wax or sealer.

Vinyl-asbestos Tile

Vinyl-asbestos tile is a full thickness of vinyl resins, plasticizers, pigments, and fillers overlaid on a backing of various regular or alkali-resistant materials. Although this type of flooring is adequate, asbestos dust is considered a cancer-producing agent.

Vinyl Tile

Homogeneous vinyl tile is composed of a full thickness of vinyl resins, plasticizers, pigments, and fillers and is formed under pressure while hot. This type of flooring is excellent for the allergic person.

Vinyl-backed Sheet or Tile

Vinyl-backed sheets or tiles have a layer composed of vinyl resins, plasticizers, pigments, and fillers overlaid on a backing of various regular or alkali-resistant materials. They are excellent products for the allergic person.

Vinyl Cork Tile

Vinyl cork tile is a full thickness of vinyl resins, plasticizers, pigments, fillers, and granulated cork and is formed under pressure while hot. This is excellent flooring for the allergic person.

Rubber Sheet and Tile

Rubber sheets and tiles are a thickness of vulcanized rubber compounded with a binder that has reinforcing fibers, pigments, and fillers. These products are satisfactory for the allergic person if they are coated with a vinyl finish.

Linoleum Sheet and Tile

Linoleum is composed of oxidized linseed oil (a flax product), resins or other oxidized oleoresinous binders mixed with ground cork, wood flour, mineral fillers, and pigments and pressed on burlap or saturated felt backing. This type of flooring has numerous allergenic sources from its dust and should be avoided by anyone who is allergic. Vinyl linoleums are suitable because these fibers are embedded in the vinyl products.

Cork Tile

Cork tile is a full thickness of compressed granulated cork bonded with a heat-processed resinous binder. This product is undesirable for the allergic person.

Rotogravure Printed Vinyl

In rotogravure printed vinyl, photographic reproductions are printed onto vinyl sheets and then coated with clear vinyl. This product is excellent for the allergic person.

Seamless Flooring

Seamless flooring is made with acrylics, urethane, epoxies, polyesters, or combinations of plastics. These floors are ideal for the allergic person. A typical floor of this type begins with a pigmented base coat such as epoxy. It is laid thickly across a clean smooth floor. While the base coat is still wet, wafer-thin plastic chips are spread onto the surface where they stick. After this dries, the chips sticking above the surface are sanded down, and then three to four clean glaze coats of urethane are applied. After drying for several hours and curing for a couple of days, the floor is finished and ready to use.

Seamless flooring provides a very low-maintenance floor if the materials have been applied correctly. It never needs waxing; it need not be scrubbed because of its nonporous surface; and it sheds dust. It has no seams to catch dirt, and it can be continued up the baseboard to eliminate a corner crevice or corner seam. It is very tough and will take roller skates and children's roughhousing without a scratch. This type of floor lasts for years and years. The success of this type of flooring depends upon the initial proper application. Once the floor is laid down, it cannot be removed.

Wood Floors

A floor finished with a Swedish floor finish or polyurethane will last for years before the finish will wear down to the wood. These floors have a high shine and will retain the gloss for a long time. Although heavy foot traffic will eventually dull the finish, the protection from exposure to the wood will remain for a long time. Carefully selected waxes can be used to preserve the finish longer. A wet mop can be used on these finishes, which makes them ideal.

Carpet and Carpet Padding

If you feel you want to carpet the home, careful selection of the type of weave and the fiber can make it a good choice if you have a good vacuum system.

Basically short, single-level looped, densely constructed carpets are best. Various patterns recommended include sculptured patterns, one-level pile or a combination of cut and uncut short loops called tip-sheared, all cut pile called velvet, short loop or cut pile, and random sheer or very tightly woven carpets. The long shags and loops harbor too much dust to make them worth the work to keep them clean. See the following chart for suggested carpet fibers.

Good carpet padding will give resiliency, absorb noise, make vacuum cleaning more efficient, act as an insulator against heat and cold, and will protect the carpet from wear and tear. Padding made of hair, hair and fiber, or rubberized hair and fiber is not recommended. These pads are sources for animal fibers, are dust-making sources, and are susceptible to mildew.

CARPET PADDING

MATERIAL	PRINCIPAL TRAITS
Sponge Rubber	
Flat	Persons sensitive to chemicals may be bothered by odor during first months after installation.
Waffled	In some cases molded in clay forms. Unless washed thoroughly of this clay, it may become a dust-making source as padding gets old.
Foam Rubber	
Flat	Compresses more than sponge, but recovers just as fast.
Waffled	Clay products can be a problem.
Polyurethane	Depending on the grade, some have tendency to stay flat where heavy weight has been on them.

CARPET PADDING

— *CONTINUED* —

MATERIAL	PRINCIPAL TRAITS
Composite Foam	Particles of foam are fused together. Products used to fuse should be investigated to be sure animal glues were not used.

CARPET RECOMMENDATIONS

FIBER	PRINCIPAL TRAITS
Nylon	Abrasion resistant — 20 oz. or more
	High static electricity can be reduced with proper humidification of the home.
	Tends to soil in spots, but easy to clean.
	Sheen present in most brands.
	Pills and sheds when new.
Acrylic	Bulky fiber gives wool look.
	Good resilience.
	Easy to clean.
	Abrasion resistance is excellent if at least 25 oz. per square yard.
	Less pilling if the weave is tight and twisted pile. Pills when new.

CARPET RECOMMENDATIONS

— CONTINUED —

FIBER	PRINCIPAL TRAITS
Modacrylic	Principally used in blends, especially with acrylic fibers.
Polypropylene	Not as resilient as other fibers. Outstanding stain resistance. Dye problems with blues and greens. Abrasion resistant. Mildew resistant.
Polyester	Bulky fiber gives wool look. Stain resistance a mild problem. Abrasion resistant, excellent if at least 25 oz. per square yard.

FURNITURE

Furniture can be a source for allergy symptoms because of its construction, its surface, or the furniture conditioners used to clean and polish. The guideline is to purchase furniture that has a hard finish that requires only damp cleaning. This, however, does not make for a homey environment. Depending on the type of furniture you desire, the following guidelines can be implemented.

Frames and Finishes

For firm upholstered furniture, use a hard urethane block core placed between two layers of foam rubber. Coil springs are frequently encased in this center core as well.

Framing of upholstered furniture is usually wood; however, chrome steel has become popular when the designer wishes to expose the frame design. Steel tubing, webbed synthetic rubber straps, and glass fiber frames and shells are also common. Rigid polyurethane frames covered in nylon-stretch or vinyl fabrics or molded shells made of fiberglass combined with polyurethane resin or modular flexible block, and inflatable vinyl sofas and chairs are just a few of the contemporary designs that are allergen-free and suitable for easy care.

A number of laminated finishes are put onto furniture to give various appearances. These include a process whereby flexible vinyl is printed to look like wood grains and is then wrapped around wood cores in a permanent bonding. You may have seen this finish simulated as gold, silver, pewter, bronze, or some other variety. These finishes are well suited for good allergy control. Just as suited are the thermoplastic moldings that are attached to furniture to represent carved wood. Laminates made of layers of wood, plastic fabric or paper bonded together by heat and pressure, and vinyl veneers are also ideal.

Fabrics

A number of fabrics on the market are synthetic and well suited for good allergy control. Synthetic fibers need not be treated with dust retardants or soil repellants because they naturally stay clean and resist dirt. Suitable fabrics include acrylics, nylon, polyester, and a few others described below:

- ✓ **Polypropylene.** Polypropylene is stain-proof, 99.4 percent moisture-proof, non-absorbent to oil, grease, lipstick, crayon, dirt, and ink.

- ✓ **Sprayed vinyl.** Vinyl spray is applied to any fabric by the manufacturer to help resist dirt and to seal the surface.

- ✓ **Vinyl fabric.** Vinyl fabrics are soft, supple, pliable, and can simulate any fabric weave. Some are woven with nylon to resemble brocades.

- ✓ **Laminated tricot knit.** Nylon, latex foam and cotton knit backing are knit into a single layer of cloth. They are then silk-screened and then immersion-treated with a soil and stain repellant.

Rescuing Old Favorites

Sometimes you may have items that you do not want to give up but are sources for allergy symptoms. This might include a collection, antique or old furniture, or oiled woods.

In some cases, removing antique or old furniture is the only solution to allergen control. Antique and old furniture must have all the surfaces and upholstery redone if you wish to keep them. The older an item is, the more antigenic it can be. By covering all the wood surfaces with a plastic coating, you will seal these dust and mold sources. This sealing includes the inside of the furniture as well.

If you have upholstered furniture that cannot be replaced at this time, remove animal or plant fibers and use polyurethane or one of the recommended fillers for the interior. Beneath chairs, sofas, day beds, and so on, tack a plastic or nonporous sheeting over the entire surface to restrict the dust-making sources to the interior of the item. Treat all fabric surfaces that are not synthetic with Dust Seal or Allergex every six months.

If you love oiled woods and cannot give them up, there is really no adequate solution except to find a highly refined furniture conditioner that does not give off gas. Many of these conditioners are oils from allergenic plants such a linseed or flax. You might find that you can make your own lemon oil with household oils that you are not allergic to.

Whatever you collect, if it hung on a wall or placed around the room, it will become a source for dust. Collections can be placed behind glass frames or in enclosed cabinets with glass doors. This includes stuffed game, dolls, or any soft cloth item.

WINDOW TREATMENT

Draperies or curtains are not recommended because of their dust-holding capability. A few types of window treatments that might be used to replace drapes and curtains are laminated shades, woven wood shades, shoji screens, vertical blinds, miniblinds, and shutters with a smooth, hard finish or with fiberglass inserts.

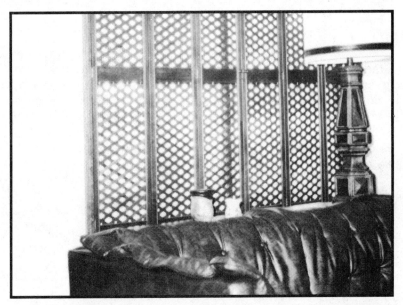

Window Treatment for Living Room. This window has been covered with an unusual shutter with a smooth furniture finish. It can be wiped with a damp cloth. The leather sofa is also suitable for good allergy control.

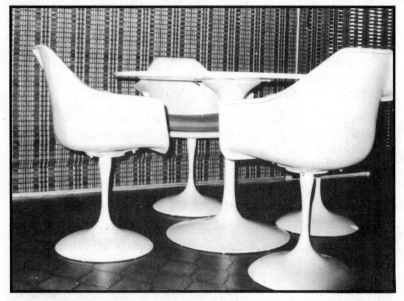

The ideal dinette. The vinyl floor, woven woods and molded dinette set make this room ideal for good allergy control.

WALLS

In the chapter on building, the different paints that are desirable for someone who is allergic were described. Paint, however, is not the only wall treatment the allergic person can have in the home. Many other methods for decorating walls can be used. In fact, the variety of smooth-textured wall surfaces is so great that there is no reason why the home should ever look like a clinic.

Vinyl Wall Coverings

Three categories of vinyl wall papers are recommended for the allergic person's home. Plastic-coated wallpaper is ordinary wallpaper with a coating of vinyl. This paper can be damp-wiped but is considered fragile compared to other types of vinyl coverings. Vinyl-latex-impregnated paper has been laminated to lightweight woven cloth and then coated with vinyl plastic. This type can be scrubbed and can take normal day-to-day wear

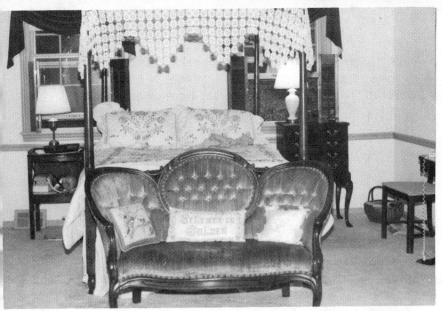

This room is a problem. The antique furniture has not been sealed inside and underside. Velvet window treatment, flax-filled pillows on settee, and sisal-filled settee will all produce dust. Goose-down bed pillows are not encased as well as the mattress and box springs. The canopy is old cotton; carpet is wool; and settee upholstery is old velvet — all materials will break down to form dust. Dust balls will be found under this bed.

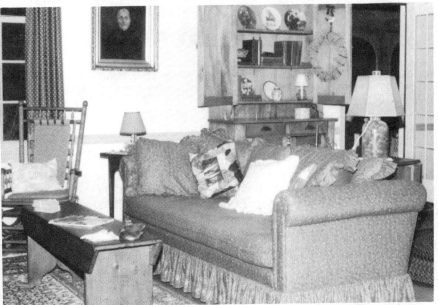

The style of furniture makes no difference in controlling allergens. Antique furniture should be sealed on all inside and underside surfaces. A hard-smooth, outer finish is ideal as long as waxes are avoided. In this picture, all pillows and the sofa have been filled with dacron. Pillow covers can be taken off and cleaned. Although curtains or drapes are not recommended, these can be cleaned frequently. The window and sofa fabric are very tight-weave cotton with a finish on them. Hardwood floor is sealed and can be damp wiped. The area carpet can be cleaned frequently.

without damage. Polyvinyl chloride is the best covering. Chloride resin acts as a binder, which is laminated to a lightweight woven cloth of polyester or rayon. Heavy grades of this wall-covering will take unusually severe use. Some even can be used as upholstery.

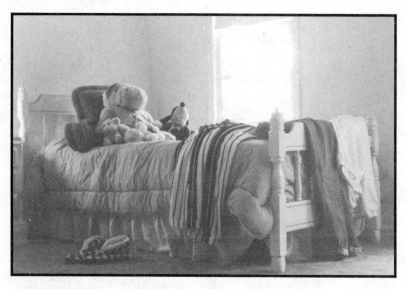

Clutter is ok. Actually, this room is very well suited for good allergy control. Stuffed toys and bedrest are filled with dacron. All bedding and clothing on the bed are washable. Mattress, box springs, and pillow are encased with the recommended zippered encasings. The carpet is ideal.

They are especially suitable for family rooms and children's rooms.

All three of these wall coverings are available as adhesive-backed papers or prepasted papers. Adhesive-backed coverings are backed with a pressure-sensitive adhesive that fastens the covering firmly in place. The prepasted types merely require wetting and then can be applied to the wall. The adhesive and prepasted wall coverings are especially desirable because they eliminate exposures to adhesives when you apply them yourself. Also, wheat paste, commonly used in the past, must be avoided because it harbors mold and eventually decomposes to become a great source of allergens.

Vinyl wallpapers resist mildew, stains, and alcohol, and they are moth-proof. Standard wallpapers without vinyl coatings are not advised for the allergic person. Wallpaper that is not vinyl or vinyl-coated can be treated with one of the products that seal the surface.

Other wall treatments that might be considered include metal tiles, mirrors, cork squares that are sealed with vinyl, and plastic panels. Ceramic tiles with silicone-sealed grout are also suitable. Hardboard panels should be investigated carefully before purchased. The composite types are bound with chips and glues and could bring a problem into the home. Generally the vinyl-coated panels are well suited for good allergy control.

9 ET CETERA—SPECIAL PEOPLE, SPECIAL PLACES

For people who are allergic, comprehensive efforts to keep their lives in balance require paying special attention to certain situations. Vacations, pets, and hospitalizations are just a few examples.

PETS

People who are allergic should not have furry or feathered pets in the home. Animals are constantly shedding their dander, which will penetrate the entire house and become a part of the housedust. Even if the animal is removed from the home, it may take many weeks before the dander can be eliminated completely. Until carpet and upholstery are replaced, dander will remain.

Caged Furred Pets

If a pet is allowed to run outdoors, pollen, molds, and dust can be present in the coat when the animal comes indoors. When these allergens are carried into the home, they become part of the household air. For this reason, caged pets are preferred over other animals, but they are not recommended.

Obviously, a caged pet should not be obtained if the potential owner or other occupant of the home has a known allergy to the pet. The cage must be carefully maintained to discourage molds and bacteria. The cage must not be in the bedroom.

Feathered Pets

A bird with its constant fluttering tends to spread feather dust into the air. The home is then filled with this dust, no matter how small the bird may be. Also molds and bacteria flourish in a bird cage.

Ideal Pets

Tropical fish, turtles, lizards, snakes, toads, frogs, salamanders, and insects such as ants are examples of pets that disperse nothing into the atmosphere. These pets are ideal for the allergic person's household.

If you have a mild allergy to your furred or feathered pet, your physician may suggest that you keep the animal outside if possible. If keeping the pets outside cannot be considered, try sending it to a friend's home for a few weeks to see if your allergy symptoms get better while the pet is away. You can visit the pet during this test period, and the time will provide a transition if the pet must stay out of the home.

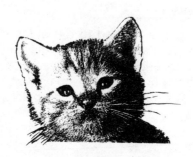

Special Situations

If you absolutely will not remove a pet from the home, a few products are available that can be used to retard the dander and reduce the possibility of allergy symptoms. Most physicians feel that removing the pet is necessary, and they do not favor such treatment of the animal. By all means, do not allow the animal in the bedroom even if it is treated.

If you are a horse owner, do not groom and spend time around the animal in the stable. However, you might try riding in an area away from the stables. The clothing worn for riding should be stored separately, away from other clothing and out of the bedroom.

HOSPITALIZATIONS

Some allergic people normally do well in maintaining good control of their allergic symptoms but end up having allergy problems when they are admitted to a hospital. Frequently it pays to be a fussy patient even if doing so may mean postponing a hospital visit. The hospital staff may consider you a selfish eccentric, but you are the one with the problem...and you should insist upon certain specifications for your stay.

Ask the admitting office to put you in a private room or with a patient who does not smoke or who does not have a large number of visitors. Visitors frequently wear perfume or smoke. Ask the admitting office to find out if any painting or remodeling is going on around the room scheduled for you. Check to see if a janitor's closet is near your room; it might contain cleaning agents that may annoy you.

Usually hospital rooms are well suited for good control of the environment. Occasionally, drapes or upholstered furniture may be dusty, but, as a rule, they should not be a problem.

When you go to the hospital, take your own unscented toiletry products rather than using the articles furnished by the hospital. If you have food allergy, contact the dietitian to check your meals for ingredients you should be avoiding.

Your allergist should know that you are going to be hospitalized so that medications you may be taking can be checked for potential reactions. Essentially, your fate is up to you. It is hoped that physicians and medical staff personnel will eventually be trained to be more sensitive to the needs of the allergic patient.

VACATIONS AND RECREATION

For the allergic person, a good vacation can be ruined because of sensitivities to a location, foods, or elements of a recreational activity. You do not have to remain in the protected environment of your home. However, to enjoy life, some careful planning is recommended. Vacations can and should be a pleasure.

Going to Camp

As long as the physician says it is permissible for a child to attend camp, the child should be allowed to go. By the time they are old enough to go to camp, allergic children should be responsible enough to recognize the things they need to avoid. Just before going to camp, the child should be checked by the physicians and given medications and instructions for the camp nurse.

The Asthma and Allergy Foundation offers publications on camps for children who have allergies and asthma. Some of the programs are geared to help children take responsibility for their health, to learn how to live with their restrictions, and to enjoy a successful first time away from the protected environment of home.

Outdoor Camping

Nowadays, the locale and its pollen sources, the food to be eaten, and the gear to be used can all be controlled. If you select an outdoor camping location and a time that is not in a pollen season that will bother you, pack food you can eat, and use the newer camping gear, your trip should be a success.

The newer camping materials tend to be synthetic. Sleeping bags filled with dacron and tents made with synthetics are all to the advantage of the allergic person. Chilling or excessive heat can be alleviated by several protective garment materials that are designed to shield a person from extremes in weather conditions. The new dry meals can be tested before you go on your trip, so you will know which ones you can eat.

Campers or Motor Homes and Trailers

An ideal way to ensure the lowest possible exposures to allergens is to take your lodging with you. The present campers, motor homes, or trailers are ideally suited for good allergy control. Only minor modifications are required.

Like the home, the decorative fibers and materials can cause trouble. However, the new plastic or plastic-coated interiors are excellent because they can be kept clean and do not serve as a dust-making or mold-harboring source for allergy. Bedding should be no problem if you follow the same suggestions that you use for your bedroom at home.

Lodges and Hotels

Unfortunately, it is a hazard for allergic people to travel around the country when they must rely on lodges or hotels. As a guideline to a better trip, try the following:

- ✦ Request hotels that offer "no smoking" floors. (Hotel chains that advertise no smoking accommodations include Best Western, Hilton, Holiday Inns, Howard Johnson, Hyatt, Marriott, Quality International, Ramada, Sheraton, TraveLodge and Westin. Call their 800 numbers to make your request.)

- ✦ Request hotels that do not allow pets.

- ✦ Avoid old historic hotels.

- ✦ Avoid brand new hotels, but seek out newer ones for your stay.

- ✦ Seek hotels off busy freeways and away from industry.

Hay Fever Holiday

For those who wish to take a vacation from hay fever, selection of the vacation spot must be careful. Generally, coastal areas that sit in the ocean breezes are a good choice. A winter holiday in the snow is another safe choice, as is a vacation in the mountains in the fall, winter, and early spring before the pollen season. If you have not lived in the desert, chances are you will not be sensitive to the pollens there. In Chapter 3 on allergens, the pollen seasons and locales are listed. Use this guide to plan a hay-fever-free holiday. Other reference sources are listed at the end of the book.

Transportation

As more and more people give up smoking, airlines may begin to restrict smoking in all of the airplane. Three airlines in Hawaii, Aloha, Hawaiian Air and Mid-Pacific Air, run non-smoking flights. Northwest does not allow smoking on all domestic flights.

Thrifty Rent-A-Car and Elite Rent-A-Car reserve some cars for non-smokers. Use their 800 numbers to make your request. Trains are also introducing restrictions on smoking. Amtrak reserves entire cars for non-smokers. On some schedules smoking is allowed in certain cars: others restrict smoking in lounge and dining cars and permit cigar smoking in sleeping quarters only.

A few simple measures can be used to make the family automobile allergy-free. When purchasing the automobile, select an air conditioning system that allows for "inside" air circulation with cooled and normal air temperature. This allows for inside circulation of air when you are traveling through pollen areas, heavy air pollution, or other areas that potentially might expose you to allergens. A note of caution — inside circulation for a long period of time without some air exchange with the outdoor air may be dangerous if you have a carbon monoxide leak. Animals should not be allowed to ride in the car. If they do, the vehicle should be vacuumed thoroughly after the trip. Sometimes molds develop in the tubes that connect the air-conditioning system to the car's interior. If you notice a musty odor, circulate heat through the air-conditioning system for a few minutes. In humid climates, this should be done once a week. As long as the car is kept vacuumed and clean, it should not be a source of allergy symptoms.

HOLIDAYS

For the allergic person, the holidays can result in symptoms. Most of these are related to ingestion of unusual foods; however, some other sources not commonly thought of as allergens or irritants may be the culprits.

HOLIDAYS—
SOME COMMON SOURCES FOR ALLERGY

Valentine's Day	Chocolate and other candies Dyes in candy
Easter	Chocolate and other candies Dyes in candy Perfume Early spring pollens (grasses)
Memorial Day	Late spring and early summer pollens
July 4th	Firework smoke Summer pollens (trees) Foods - in season
Labor Day	Late summer pollens (weeds)
Halloween	Molds Chocolate and candies Dyes
Thanksgiving	Mixed nuts Eggnog Spices Foods not usual to the diet Molds
Christmas	Mixed nuts Eggnog Spices Foods not usual to the diet Decorations taken out of storage Christmas tree—tree releases pollens as it dries; flocking on the tree; coloring sprayed on the tree.

STINGING INSECTS

If you know you are allergic to stinging insects, your physician has probably given you an avoidance sheet, along with an emergency kit in case you are stung. As review, the highest risk from stinging insects will be in a garden, around feeding grounds such as garbage cans, water, flowers, and orchards with ripe fruit, and picnic areas.

Some guidelines for protection include:

- Wear shoes at all times.
- Wear dark clothes that are not loose and that cover your arms and legs.
- Do not wear scented toiletry products (soaps, perfumes, etc.).
- Avoid rapid movements.
- Keep your car closed and use the air conditioner.
- Use screens for your home.
- When eating or cooking outdoors, keep food covered until eaten.
- Use insecticides around the patio, garbage area, or places that attract insects.
- Keep an aerosol insecticide in your car for emergency use.
- Carry your emergency kit with you at all times.
- Don't do outdoor sports or activities alone.

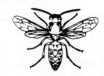

SCHOOL

School represents a large portion of a child's day. Therefore, it is worth checking the school for potential problems if your child is coming home ill.

The following are common sources for causing allergy symptoms:

- ✓ Sleeping on the carpet during rest time
- ✓ Irritating cleaning products
- ✓ Art classes
- ✓ Woodworking classes
- ✓ Chalk dust (may irritate)
- ✓ Gym dressing room (mold may be present)
- ✓ Printing class
- ✓ Library (old books are dusty)
- ✓ Furred or feathered animals in the classroom
- ✓ Painting of the building or other renovations done during school time
- ✓ Exercise during the times when the level of air pollution is high
- ✓ Old furniture, carpets, or drapes
- ✓ Storerooms that contain papers, magazines, or chemicals
- ✓ Forced-air heating and air-conditioning system may spread dust or molds

The Washington, D. C., chapter of the Asthma and Allergy Foundation has developed policy and further information on how to handle problems that allergic children may have at school.

MOVING

Everyone makes changes in living locations from time to time. The allergic person may find a new location good or bad, depending on a number of factors.

The stress of making a major change can upset your physical balance, and with new environmental exposures, the physical balance can be upset even more.

Climates and geographical changes can create a problem. Moving to a new geographical location might bring about a feeling of well-being for some time. It takes approximately two years for the body to acquire new allergies. It may be that during a third year at the new location, you will have a recurrence of allergy symptoms. A new allergy evaluation may be necessary to determine if your allergies to pollens or molds have changed.

The interior environment can be different despite moving all of your personal belongings. The materials used in construction and decoration of the home may be sources of allergy. The following guidelines can be used when purchasing a home is not planned or modifications on a rented home are not permitted.

RENTAL GUIDE CHECKLIST

Location

_____ The home should not have damp walls or roof leaks.

_____ The home should be located away from busy traffic and freeways.

_____ The home should be located away from industrial pollutants.

_____ The home should not be downwind from cultivated farmland, wetlands, grain elevators, golf courses, or grassy fields if pollens or molds are a serious problem.

RENTAL GUIDE CHECKLIST

Home Interior

_____ Wall surfaces should be smooth and washable.

_____ Waterbase or latex paints should be used on walls, ceilings and woodwork. Avoid oil-base paints.

_____ The ceiling surface should be smooth and washable. If an acoustical ceiling over 15 years old is present, it should be sealed with latex base paint.

_____ Vinyl sheet flooring or vinyl tiles require no waxes and are considered ideal.

_____ Asphalt tiles or floors of wood should be sealed with acrylic floor sealer.

_____ Carpet can be considered if it is 100 percent synthetic and includes a synthetic foam pad.

_____ If a previous occupant had a dog or cat, do not rent the home.

— CONTINUED —

_____ Check to see if the owner or manager will permit removal of curtains or drapes. Cover the windows with one of the materials suggested in the chapter on decorating. Because this is usually not practical unless the owner or manager will provide the changes, the curtains or drapes should be cleaned according to the cleaning schedule in the chapter on home control. An alternative is to create a drape with sheets that can be washed frequently.

_____ The windows should close tightly.

_____ Electric heat is ideal. Use special filters if the home has forced air heating.

_____ There should be no plumbing leaks.

SOURCES OF COMMON ALLERGENS

Foods, Pollens, Molds and Environmentals

The following index has been prepared as a guide for the avoidance of allergenic sources. Avoiding every allergen that you test positive to makes life too complicated. Your physician will recommend what allergens you should avoid according to your history, tests, and the severity of your allergy symptoms.

ACACIA GUM
See Vegetable Gums

ALCOHOLIC BEVERAGES
Bourbon • corn, rye, wheat, barley malt, mineral water, yeast
Gin • distilled from rye and other grains and flavored with juniper berries, cinnamon and coriander seeds
Rum • distilled from cane sugar
Tequila • cactus
Vodka • distilled from wheat, rye, potatoes
Wine • fermented juice of grapes and fruits
Whiskey • distilled from fermented mash of various grains, especially rye, wheat, corn, barley

ALDER
Alder, Birch, *Hazelnut* Family (*Betulaceae*)
Pollen found in the Rocky Mountains; cross sensitivity may result with all three.

ALGAE
Found in the outdoor air in certain areas of the country; seasonal variation.

ALTERNARIA
Found in outdoor air especially in humid weather; seasonal variations; found in water or damp places including pond scum.

ALMOND
Also see *Plum* Family
Nuts • found in ice cream, candy, as a dressing or as an accent for flavoring on pastry, fish, and vegetable dishes
Oil • pits of almonds, peaches, cherries that have been fermented and distilled, flavoring

AMARANTH
Amaranth (*Amaranthaceae*) is also called pigweed or waterhemp. Pollen occurs from midsummmer to September in North America. Weeds include western waterhemp, pigweed, carelessweed.
Recently amaranth has been promoted as a substitute for tobacco growers. Its uses have not been fully developed beyond cereals and flour.

ANISEED
See *Parsley* Family
Foods • chewing gum, herbs and spices, liqueurs, Chinese dishes, gin

APPLE Family
Apple, pear, crabapple, quince

APPLE
See *Apple* Family
Foods • apple butter, apple juice, cider vinegar, applejack, pectin (jellies and gumdrops), imitation flavoring (contains apple oil with cornstarch and citric acid), pectin in Turkish paste

ARROWROOT
Foods • broths, bouillon, milk as a thickener, biscuits, arrowroot cookies and cakes, puddings, and jellies

ASPERGILLUS
Mold found on food; found as mildew in dusty damp basements, bedding, and storage areas

ASPIRIN (*acetylsalicylic acid*)
See Salicylates

AVOCADO
See *Laurel* Family
Foods • green goddess salad dressing, chip dip, Mexican food as a topping, salads

BANANA
Foods • used raw in salads, flavoring for breads, cakes, cookies, ice cream

BARLEY
Foods • cereals, soups, broths, beer, ale, porter, stout, malted drinks, gin, whiskey, scotch

BEAN
See *Pea* Family
Foods • frequently found in vegetable soups, salads, and casseroles, Mexican foods

BEECH Family
Beech, chestnuts, oak Family (*Fagaceae*)
Food • beechnuts, chestnuts usually found labeled
Tree Pollen • beech, oak, chestnut, chinquapins

BEEF
If a person is sensitive to mammalian meats, he or she can usually tolerate fowl or fish.
Sources • usually obvious or labeled

BEETS
See *Goosefoot* Family
Foods • salads, preserves, beet sugar
Other Sources • pollens from many weeds belong to the *Goosefoot* Family (People sensitive to these pollens may find they cannot eat beets during the pollinating season.)

BIRCH
Alder, birch, hazelnut Family (*Betulaceae*)
Tree pollen most prominent in northeastern United States and Canada; cross sensitivity is common.

BOOKS/NEWSPAPERS/MAGAZINES
Sources • fresh printer's ink, dyes used in printing, glue used in binding, sizing, the filler in the paper, dust from sitting in storage for more than a few months.

BOTRYTIS
Fungi (mold) belonging to *Moniliaceae* Family

BUCKWHEAT
See *Buckwheat* Family
Food • pancakes, cereals, and bakery goods

BUCKWHEAT Family
Weeds • sheep sorrel, curlydock, bitterdock, buckwheat
Food • rhubarb

CAMEL
Sources • mixed with wool, blankets, overcoats, felt hats, rugs, carpets, hair brushes, paint brushes

CASTOR BEAN
Castor Bean Family (*Euphorbiaceae*), cultivated in Southern United States
Medical • castor oil
Cosmetics • lipstick (including some hypo-allergenic brands), hair creams
Other Sources • fertilizers, used in the manufacturing of artificial leather, lubricant for engines, found in varnishes and paints, soaps, typewriter ink, candles; people living near castor bean processing plant may inhale particles from the air

CAFFEINE
Probably a pharmacologic effect rather than allergy;
Sources • found in APC, Exedrin, Coriciden, cola drinks, coffee, tea, chocolate

CAT
Cat Family includes lion, tiger, lynx, leopard, panther
Sources • pelts and trimming, cat dander. Even though a cat is removed from the home, the furniture may contain hair and dander for many months.

CARROT
See *Parsley* Family
Foods • soups, salads, combination dishes, decorative accent with entrees
Other Sources • relationship to carotene dyes; carotene is added to yeast for Vitamin A

CASHEW
Cashew Family
Food • candy, ice cream, main dishes

CELERY
Parsley Family
Foods • mixed vegetable juices, Chinese dishes, salads, celery flavor in soups, salads, and combination dishes

CHAETOMIUM
Fungi (mold) belonging to the *Zygomycetes* Family

CHENOPODIACEAE
Goosefoot Family includes saltbush (*Atriplex*), smother weed (*Bassia*), sugar beet (*Beta*), goosefoot, pigweed (*Chenopodium*), burning bush (*Kochia*), Russian thistle (*salsola*); cross reaction may occur between this Family and the *Amaranth* Family; most common in the western United States

CHICKEN
Foods • It is possible to be sensitive to all fowl, and eggs. Other sources • feathers found in pillows, mattresses, furniture, feather decorations in clothing, and the home

CHICLE
See Vegetable Gums
Source • chewing gum

CHOCOLATE
See Vegetable Gums
See Caffeine
Cross reactions to cola nut are possible; therefore, cola drinks may cause symptoms.
Foods • used as flavoring in many foods and usually labeled.

CITRUS Family
Orange, lemon, grapefruit, tangerine, lime, limequat, kumquat, citron, bergamot (perfumes)
Foods • citron—oil of citronella in candies, preserves, cakes, puddings, and oil of citrus used in pectin

CLADOSPORIUM
Fungi (mold) belonging to *Dematiaceae* Family. Also called *Hormodendrum*; found as a seasonal mold in the air.

COCONUT
Palm Family
Foods • milk substitutes, grated in cakes, frostings, candies, desserts, in oils labeled "vegetable oil," margarines, coconut milk, Polynesian main dishes and drinks
Cosmetics • hair rinses, shampoos, suntan lotions and oils

CODFISH
Vitamin preparations containing "natural" ingredients, vitamins labeled codfish oil, seafood dishes

COFFEE
Foods • flavoring in ice cream, candy and bakery products; instant and regular coffee
(If there are allergy symptoms, it may be the coffee additives —chicory, cereals, chestnuts, legumes, carrots, or coffee substitutes may include dates, okra seeds, chicory, beechnuts, horse chestnuts, asparagus seeds, dried figs, cereal grains.)

COMPOSITE FAMILY
Flowers • sunflower, dahlia, chrysanthemum, pyrethrum
Weeds • giant ragweed, short ragweed, southern ragweed, western ragweed, slender ragweed, cocklebur, sagebrush, mugwort, wormwood,
Foods • lettuce, oyster plant, salsify, chicory, endive

CORN AND CORN PRODUCTS
Foods
    Beverages • ale, beer, carbonated drinks, bourbon, whiskies, instant coffee, fruit juices, gin, liquors, soy bean milk, instant tea

Desserts • baking mixes, baking powders, bleached wheat flours, vanilla, breads, pastries, cakes, cookies, confectioners sugar, cornstarch, cream pies, cream puffs, puddings, frostings, gelatin, custards, sherbets, ice creams, sundaes

Main Dishes and Accompaniments • batters for frying, catsup, cheese, chili, chop suey, corn flakes, gravies, soups, sauces, salad dressings, graham crackers, hams, jellies, bacon, bologna, luncheon meat, tamales, enchiladas, monosodium glutamate, margarine, peanut butter, canned vegetables, popcorn, preserves, coated rice, sandwich spreads, syrups

Cosmetics and Toiletry products • body powders, bath powders, dental powders and cleaners, talcum, toothpaste, soap

Medical uses • aspirin, filler in pills, gelatin capsules, vitamins, glucose, lozenges, ointments, suppositories, dextrose, cough syrup

Other Sources • adhesives for envelopes, stamps, stickers, tape, ironing starch, paper containers, boxes, cups, plates, and paper food wrappers that may be coated with cornstarch

COTTONSEED

See *Malvacea* Family

Food • cereals, oil labeled "vegetable," shortening, margarine, mayonnaise, canned fish packed in cottonseed oil, fried foods, potato chips, doughnuts, chocolate and confection candy, olive and other oils may include cottonseed, polished fruit

Medical • camphorated oil, as an oil base to liquid medicines, liniments, creams, and castor oil

Cosmetic • lipsticks, perfume, creams, oil base lotions, creams, suntan products

Other Sources • cotton linters (during the process of harvesting cotton, long fibers, called linters, are removed), fabrics, bedding, upholstery, rugs, wadding or batting for pads and cushions, wet varnishes, waterproofing, paint, fertilizers, feed for cattle, poultry, horses, hogs, sheep, dogs

COW

Foods • beef, cow's milk

Other Sources • hair used in oxite rug pads, brushes, felt, blankets, fur toy animals, insulation, clothing of people working around cows: i.e., dairy farm, cattle ranch

CUCUMBER
See *Gourd* Family
Foods • pickles, salads, vegetable dishes, appetizer

DATE
See *Palm* Family
Foods • baked goods, candies, wines, date oil may be included in "vegetable" oils, date flour

DERRISROOT
Sources • insecticides (rotenone)

DOG
Sources • dog hair is combined with wool to make Chinese rugs; used in hair pads; dog hair and dander remain for long periods of time in furnishings after removal from a home; a person not sensitive to dog may be reacting to pollens or molds in the dog's hair.

EGGS
A cross reaction to chicken, chicken feathers or chicken meat may occur.
Foods (cooked or raw)
> **Baked Goods** • cake, cookies, doughnuts, macaroons, pastries, batters, pretzels, french toast, pie crust, muffins, prepared flours, meringues
>
> **Frozen Desserts** • ice cream, sherbets
>
> **Sauces/Cream Mixtures** • mayonnaise, hollandaise, tartar, salad dressing, icings, fondue, chocolate creams, filled candy bars, glazed pastry, puddings
>
> **Beverages** • ovaltine, ovomalt, rootbeer
>
> **Prepared flours**
>
> **Meats** • sausage, meatloaf and casseroles; consomme and some wines are cleared with egg

Cosmetic • hair shampoos, rinses
Medical • vaccines may be cultured in eggs, pharmaceutical emulsions, laxatives
Other Sources • egg albumen used in photography, in printing on cotton, tanning and other leather preparations

ENGLISH PLANTAIN
Plantain Family (*Plantaginaceae*), found throughout the United States especially the eastern and western coasts; common weed found in lawns and open areas

EPICOCCUM
Fungi (mold) belonging to the *Tuberculariaceae* Family; found in households

EUCALYPTUS
Eucalyptus Family (*Myrtaceae*) includes bottlebrushes; pollen tends to be bee pollinated; therefore, not significant to allergy; however, some of these trees have a strong odor that may cause symptoms.

FEATHERS
Sources • (duck and goose most common) pillows, mattresses; overstuffed furniture, clothing, home and clothing decorations, zoo, circus, stuffed birds in home or office

FISH
Sturgeon, sardine, trout, shad, pike, tuna, sunfish, snapper, sole, scrod, caviar, herring, salmon, eel, pickerel, bluefish, bass, porgy, halibut, haddock, anchovy, smelt, whitefish, carp, mackerel, swordfish, perch, flounder, codfish

Food • any of the above fresh or canned (fish may be canned in oils causing the sensitivity rather than fish); caviar may be different kinds of fish eggs; fish oil may be used in vitamin preparations; odor of fish cooking may cause symptoms in very sensitive people.

Other Sources • fish glue may be found in old furniture, wood framing.

FLAXSEED (Also called LINSEED)
Foods • cereals, flaxseed tea, milk from cows eating flaxseed meal, muffins

Cosmetics and Toiletries • wave setting preparations, shampoos, hair tonics, depilatories

Medical • laxatives

Other Sources • patent leather, electrical insulating material, fabric using flax fibers, upholstered furniture, mattresses, cattle and poultry feed, household products, dog and cat food, furniture polish, paints, varnishes, printers' ink, carron oil, linoleum, lemon oil products, linseed oil, soaps, twine and rope, cigarette paper, Bible paper, bird lime, fiberboard, garment interlining, canvas, saddlery and leather goods sewed with flax, linen — clothing, table covers, art, damask, sheeting, towels, lampshades; oil cloth, sailcloth, wax paper

FOWL

Chicken, duck, goose, turkey, guinea hen, pigeon, pheasant, partridge, grouse

FUR

The Federal Fur Products Labeling Act requires identifying furs along these guidelines:

Beaver • brown, dense, short-length fur is often dyed and bleached

Chinchilla • dense, silky fur with grayish-blue hair

Ermine • from species of the weasel that grows a pure white coat in the winter; coat retains its non-winter brown called summer ermine.

Fox • long and glossy hair dyed in many colors besides its natural silver, white, blue and red

Lamb • five broad categories of pelts used for furs: broadtail, mouton, Persian, curly and moire

Mink • soft, lightweight, yet dense fur has soft feel; wild mink is trapped in natural habitat; ranch mink is raised under controlled conditions; mutant minks are domesticated and bred for coat color.

Muskrat • used in its natural brown and is also dressed and dyed to simulate more expensive furs

Rabbit • silky texture and is often dyed to simulate beaver, chinchilla, seal, ermine and leopard

Sable • soft, dense, medium-long fur

Seal • two classified groups, fur seal and hair seal; fur seal, from Alaska, has velvety texture and the fur is straightened, finished and dyed; hair seal has short, shiny fur that is more like coarse hair than fur.

Squirrel • gray skins are used without dying; most squirrel is dyed to different shades.

Spotted furs • jaguar, leopard, spotted cat and ocelot are difficult to distinguish.

FUSARIUM

Fungi (mold) found in the air and spreads by rain drops

GLUE

Animal or Fish Glue. Since synthetic glues are used more and more, the animal or fish glues are not too common.

Sources • found in old furniture, old books, woodworking, paper industry products in labels and envelopes; imported silk fabrics frequently contain fish glues that do not get washed out of the fabric.

GOAT

Allergy to goat may result in reaction to goat milk.

Foods • goat milk, foreign cheeses

Other Sources • cashmere, bedding, upholstered furniture, fur coats, shoes, muffs, angora, rugs, cushions, robes, braids, trim, mohair, shaving brushes, gloves, wigs, alpaca yarns

GOOSEFOOT FAMILY

Also called chenopods

Weeds • russian thistle (tumbleweed), lambquarters, salt bush

Foods • beet, spinach, swiss chard

GOURD FAMILY

Cantaloupe, casaba, cucumber, honeydew, pumpkin, squash, watermelon, muskmelon, Persian, crenshaw

GRAPE FAMILY

Foods • wild and cultivated grapes found in juices and jellies; grape seed oil used in salad oil and resembles olive oil; raisins; wines (Note: allergy to wine may be due to sulfides, yeasts, or as a chemical reaction to old red wines); cognac; grape vinegar; Greek dishes.

GRAPEFRUIT

See *Citrus* Family

Foods • fruit drinks, salads, canned and fresh fruit, as flavoring in cola drinks, spritzers, ale, gin, and prepared cake bakery mixes

Cosmetics • shampoo, hair rinses

GRASSES

Includes grasses (*Poaceae* or *Gramineae*), sedges (*Cyperaceae*) and rushes (*Juncaceae*). Grasses include redtop (*Agrostis*), vernalgrass (*Holcus*), darnel, ryegrass (*Lolium*), timothy (*Phleum*), bluegrass and June grass (*Pao*), Bermuda (*Cynodon*), Johnson and cultivated sorghum (*Sorghum*), cross sensitivity occurs. The sedges and rushes seem to be limited in exposure and away from cities; therefore, not significant for allergy.

GUINEA PIG
Pets found in schools, homes, zoos, pet stores; medical and biological labs

GUMS
Arabic (acacia), karaya (Indian), locust bean, quince, chicle, tragacanth, carobseed

Foods • fillings, candies, mustard, jello, jelly beans, ice cream, sauces, junket, processed swiss and cheddar cheese, cream cheese, whipped cream cake icing, commercial potato salad, chewing gums, gravies, wheat cakes, diabetic foods (soybean, almond wafers, pies, custards)

Cosmetics and Toiletries • lotions, shaving preparations, mouthwash, rouge, powders, denture adhesives, toothpaste, face powders, waving lotions

Medical • laxatives, emulsified mineral oils, fillers in pills, lozenges

Other Sources • cigar wrappers, printing inks, adhesives, stamps, stickers, gummed paper

HAZELNUT
Alder, Birches, *Hazelnut* Family (*Betulaceae*); high cross sensitivity with all three

Food • found in desserts, bakery goods, as accent to main dishes

HELMINTHOSPORIUM
Fungi (mold) belonging to *Dematiaceae* Family

Source • Seasonal field molds, called corn blight, flax wilt; common mold to melons, peas, and bananas

HEMP FAMILY
Hemp, marijuana, hashish

HICKORY FAMILY
Hickory/Walnut Family (*Juglandaceae*); hickory and pecan pollen is found in eastern North America; walnut (*Juglans*) is found in the Rocky Mountains, California and Oregon.

Food • hickory and walnuts common in desserts; usually labeled in commercially prepared foods; difficult to determine in homemade or restaurant foods; walnut oil used in food preparation

HORMODENDRUM (CLADOSPORIUM)
Fungi (mold) belonging to *Dematiaceae* Family
Sources • seasonal mold found in the outdoor air and may have seasonal variation

HORSE
Sources • hairs in clothing, bedding, felt, upholstery, interlining for coats and suits, lining in shoes, fishing lines, furniture, hats, rope, hair carpet padding, mattresses, tooth and shoe brushes; found in the country, at parades, zoos, circus; an allergic person may react to the fertilizer or to people who have recently been around a horse, and clothing used for riding in a closet.

HOG
Sources • mattresses, furniture, padding, brushes, insulation, rug pads, lard

HOUSE DUST
A unique substance made up of the break-down of products of plant and animal fibers found in the home. It is not the dust that blows from outdoors. It is made up of mites, insect parts, human and animal danders

HYMENOPTERA
Stinging insects • yellow jacket, wasp, hornet, bee, fire ant

INSECTS
Includes *Hymenoptera* (bees, wasps, ants), mosquitoes, fleas, flies, cockroaches, gnats (midges)
Insect parts, decaying insects and excreta can all contribute to allergy; most significant when they swarm, especially mayflies and caddis flies.

JUTE
Made from a plant found in India
Sources • burlap, rope, sacks, baskets, rugs, mats, carpet, and carpet padding

KAPOK
Foods • vegetable oils used in cooking and salads and some margarines
Other Sources • filler for life preservers, pillow fill, mattress fill, stuffing in upholstered furniture, fabric blends

LAMB
Food • Not a common allergen; usually obvious or labeled; found in Lebanese dishes

LAUREL FAMILY
Cinnamon, bay leaves

LEGUME FAMILY (Also called *Pea* Family)
Legume Family (*Fabaceae* or *Leguminosae*) includes kidney beans, lentil, pea, soya, haricot, black eyed pea, licorice (candy, tobacco, liquors), locust bean, string bean, senna, jack bean, lima bean, navy bean, peanut, mung and acacia

Tree pollen • acacia, mimosa and mesquite trees

LILY FAMILY
Foods • asparagus, chives, garlic, leek, onion

LOBSTER
See Shellfish

Food • usually obviously labeled as lobster, fish stew

LOCUST BEAN (CAROBSEED)
Found in seeds or pods of the carob tree

Medical • antidiarrheal medications

Other sources • sizing, paper making, calico printing

MALVACEA FAMILY
Food • Okra, gumbo, cottonseed

MAPLE
Maple Family (*Aceraceae*) includes maples and box elder

MARIJUANA
See *Hemp* Family (*Cannabaceae*) includes hemps, hops and marijuana; shed abundant pollen; Illegal substance that is smoked.

MILK
Occasionally a person is sensitive to milk because of the feeds that the cow has been given such as cottonseed, grasses and weeds, or drugs such as penicillin.

Milk should be avoided in all forms. In using milk substitutes, read labels carefully and avoid "milk solids" or "casein" terminology.

Foods

　　beverages • chocolate drinks, ovaltine, evaporated or dried milk, imitation milk, fresh whole, skim, or non-fat, buttermilk;

breads • pancakes, waffles, prepared mixes, crackers, enriched breads; breaded foods • fish, vegetables, fritters, fried meats;

desserts • bakery items, pie crust, pudding, creams, mustards, junket, ice cream, milk sherbets, candies, milk chocolate;

salad dressings;

creamed dishes or casseroles • stroganoff, creamed vegetables or meat dishes, Mexican dishes (cheese);

spreads • butter, margarine, cream cheese, sour cream;

meats • hash, commercially prepared dinners or dishes, canned, frozen or dehydrated meals, bologna, weiners, frankfurters, sausages;

cheeses • all cheeses including goat milk cheeses;

sauces and gravies • white sauces, creamed gravies;

soups • canned, frozen and dehydrated cream soups;

misc. sources • foods fried in butter, yogurt, mashed potatoes, souffles, au gratin dishes, omelets, scrambled eggs

MINT FAMILY

Peppermint, spearmint, sage, rosemary, thyme

MOLD

Look up each mold by name in this index or see Chapter 3 for classification of common molds that cause allergy.

Foods • aged sour cream, sour milk, buttermilk, canned juices, crackers, breads, rye krisp, graham crackers, breads, bakery products, citrus fruits, dried fruits — raisins, pears, apricots, dates, figs, prunes, etc., cured meats; meat or fish leftovers including casseroles; saki, beer, wine, alcoholic liquors; vinegar and foods with vinegar; i.e., mayonnaise, salad dressings, catsup, chili sauce, pickles, pickled foods — beets, relishes, green olives; sauerkraut; mushrooms; vitamins; cheeses.

Household sources

Exterior	Interior
water seeping from cement foundation	homes that have been closed up for a long time i.e. summer homes/second homes/old homes
damp walls	
damp floors	homes that have antique collections
ceiling from leaks	
awnings	homes that have stuffed game collections
wet areas around the home	
barns	decorative materials i.e. wallpaper, cloth window shades, tile, tile grout
farms	
chicken/turkey houses or pens	draperies
animal corrals	upholstered furniture
underground water seepage areas	animal or plant fiber upholstery
over-watered garden areas	wood framing in furniture that has been in a flood
damp north side of home	any area of the home that has been flooded by water
fully shaded garden areas	carpet
hay bales	carpet padding (especially jute)
cut grass/weeds not cleaned from area	areas of the home that have been closed for a long period of time: closets, attic rooms, basement, forced-air-heating system, ventilators
	heating/cooling ducts that draw air from attic or beneath home

MONOSODIUM GLUTAMATE

Probably a pharmacologic effect rather than allergy

Sources • Common in Chinese dishes, and some main dish recipes

MONILIA
Fungi (mold) belonging to *Moniliaceae* Family

MORNING GLORY FAMILY
Sweet potato

MUCOR
Fungi (mold) belonging to *Zygomycetes* Family
Mold frequently found as "black" mold on bread

MULBERRY FAMILY
Mulberry Family (*Moraceae*) tends to be weedy trees or shrubs
Along with osage, orange also in the family, they can cause severe hay fever
Foods • black mulberry, fig, hops (used in beer)

MUSTARD FAMILY
Mustard Family (*Brassicaceae* or *Cruciferae*); mustard pollen in California and Oregon
Foods
Broccoli, brussels sprouts, cabbage, cauliflower, horseradish, kale, rutabaga, kohlrabi, mustard, radish, turnip, watercress

NIGHTSHADE FAMILY
Chili (*Cayenne*), eggplant, white potato, red and green peppers, tomatoes

NUTS
Walnut Family — English walnut, black walnut, butternut, black and white walnuts; see *Walnut* Family
Walnut • walnut oil used in cooking and salad oil, baked goods
Pecan • found in baked goods
Hickory • flavoring in sauces, coffee; see Walnut Family
Beechnut • used as coffee substitute, salad oil, butter substitute; see Beech
Chestnuts • flour used in bread, desserts, coffee substitute, soups, special dishes usually with chestnut in name; see Beech
Hazelnut • oil used in Russian cooking; baked goods; see Hazelnut
Other nuts that are unrelated to those above: acorn, cashew, coconut, litchi, pine

OAK

See *Beech* Family

Beeches, Chestnuts, *Oaks* (*Fagaceae*) Family

Oak trees grow throughout the United States and can cause severe hay fever.

OATS

Foods • prepared cereals usually labeled, bakery goods

Cosmetics and Toiletries • oat soap, skin lotion

OILS

Vegetable oils — cottonseed, olive, sesame, date, peanut, corn, coconut, walnut, safflower, soybean, palm

OLIVE

Ashes, olive, privet trees (*Oleaceae*); ash grows in several areas of the United States; olive and privet tend to be cultivated and are very common as ornamental plants in the southwest; olive groves are common to central California.

There is an occasional relationship between allergy to olives and olive tree pollen. A chemical is available to spray on olive trees to keep them from pollinating.

Foods • olive oil may be adulterated with cottonseed, tea seed, corn, peanut or sesame; when olive oil is used to pickle with brine and vinegar, various condiments may be allergens (fennel, laurel leaves, thyme, coriander).

Other Sources • olive oil can be found in soaps, skin conditioners.

ONION

See *Lily* Family

Foods • catsup, sauces, pickled foods, canned foods, casseroles and as an obvious ingredient to most dishes

Other sources • wild onion eaten by cows will flavor butter and milk and cause problems in highly onion-sensitive people.

ORRIS ROOT

The powder derived from the orrisroot is from drying and grinding up the plant. Oil and fine starch granules hold aromas. They are used for scents in cosmetics and toiletries. It is not as common in products as it was years ago.

Sources include: scented powders, face powders, rouge, sachets, mascara, eyebrow dye, hairsetting solutions, eye shadow, dry shampoo, lipstick, perfume, scented soaps, haircreams/tonics, facial creams, shaving creams, sunburn lotion, bath salts/powders.

PALM FAMILY

Date, coconut (*Arecaceae* or *Plamae*) Family. Date and coconut trees are cultivated commercially in Florida, California, Arizona and Hawaii; some cities in these locations use them as street plantings; pollen tends to be only around the trees and not carried in large amounts in the wind.

Food • dates, coconuts used in bakery items, alcoholic and non-alcoholic drinks; coconut oils used in margarines, vegetable oil

Cosmetics • coconut oil used in skin preparations, some cream-base cosmetics

PARSLEY FAMILY

Carrots, celery, parsley, dill, parsnip, caraway, aniseed, fennel

PEA FAMILY

See *Legume* Family

Black-eyed pea, jack bean, kidney bean, licorice, lima bean, lentil, locust bean, navy bean, pea, peanut, soya bean, string bean

PEACH

See *Plum* Family

PEANUT

See *Pea* or *Legume* Family

Foods • peanut is usually an obvious ingredient in foods; peanut oil is frequently used in salad oils labeled "vegetable oil"; used to fry foods.

PENICILLIUM

Fungi (mold) belongs to *Moniliaceae* Family

Green mold found on food; as mildew on stored items

PEPPERS

Red pepper, cayenne pepper, paprika, tabasco are found in Mexican or Italian foods.

PORK

Foods • gelatin, jello

Medical • gelatin capsules may be from pork

POTATO
See *Nightshade* Family
Food • obvious by label; casseroles, soups

PLUM FAMILY
Almond, plum-prunes, cherry, apricot, peach, nectarine

PULLARIA
Fungi (mold) belongs to *Dematiaceae* Family. Slime mold

PYRETHRUM
See *Composite* Family.
Pyrethrum is used extensively for non-toxic insecticides.
Sources • insect powders and sprays, moth-proofing, incense

QUINCE SEED
See Vegetable Gums
Sources • used as a gum in hair preparations, hand lotions, as a filler in medicines

RABBIT
See Furs for the many names that rabbit may be sold under.
Sources • found in blended fabrics such as wools, packing material, stuffing for mattresses and furniture, carpet padding, fur for lining gloves, slippers and caps, stiffening for pillows, felt hats; covering for toy animals; felts used for pianos and insulation; can be found in research labs.

RAGWEED
Ragweed, marsh-elders, and sagebrush (*Asteraceae* or *Compositae*) Family; this Family plus the grasses cause more hay fever than any other of the plants combined; there is cross sensitivity within the species.
Sources • ragweed (*Ambrosia*), marsh-elder (*Iva*), and sagebrush and wormwood (*Artemisia*) pollinate in large quantities at the end of the summer and winter in warmer climates.

RHIZOPUS
Fungi (mold) belonging to *Zygomycetes* Family
Seen as "black" mold found on breads, vegetables

RICE
Foods • Cereals, such as puffed rice, rice flakes; as prepared flours, vermicelli, macaroni, and sake.
Medical • liquid vitamin-B complex may contain rice polishings.

ROSE FAMILY
Youngberry, raspberry, blackberry, black raspberry, strawberry, loganberry, dewberry

RYE
Foods • rye bread, pumpernickel bread, knackebrod, Ry-Krisp, rye whiskey, cereals

SALICYLATES
Foods • natural salicylates include almond, apple (cider and cider vinegar), apricot, blackberries, cherries, cloves, cucumber and pickles, currants, gooseberries, grapes or raisins (wine, wine vinegar), mint flavors, nectarines, oranges, peaches, plum or prunes, raspberries, strawberries, tea, tomatoes, oil of wintergreen, bell peppers
Medical • labeled as aspirin, acetylsalicylic
Other sources • artificial colors and flavors, toothpaste, toothpowder, perfume

SEAWEED
Foods • jellies, ice cream, diabetic foods
Medical • laxatives

SHEEP
See wool, lamb

SHELLFISH
Crab, crayfish, lobster, shrimp
Shellfish are frequently a source for a very severe form of allergy symptoms. Therefore, all shellfish should be avoided if one is known to cause symptoms.

SHRIMP
See Shellfish
Foods • found in seafood dishes, as soup and is usually an obvious ingredient.

SILK
The silkworm cocoon is composed of fibers that are glued together. Some of the glue remains in the fabric after washing. Fabrics frequently have a slight scent from fish glue.
Sources • thread, fabric, clothing, silk-screen printing process, stuffing for pillows, quilts and other bedding, furniture upholstery, rugs, curtains, underwear

SORREL DOCK

Dock or sorrel (*Polygonaceae*) are weeds that pollinate about the same time as grass; dock (*Rumex*), mountain sorrel (*Oxyria*) species are wind-dispersed.

SOYBEAN

See *Legume* Family

Foods • bakery goods, sauces, candies, ice cream, soy nuts, vegetable oil, cereals, margarine/butter substitutes, milk substitutes, sausage, luncheon meats, soups, Chinese dishes, as a food additive to prevent drying in baked goods, candies and to emulsify fats, Tofu (Doufu), beer, miso (fermented soybean paste), tempeh (a fermented soybean cake), mayonnaise, shortening, salad dressing

Medical • topical skin preparations, glycerine, massage creams

Other Sources • varnish, printing ink, candles, celluloid, linoleum, paper finishes, automobile interior plastics, upholstery fabric, rubber substitute, textile fabrics, fertilizer, plywood adhesive, artificial petroleum, oilcloth, lubrication oil, enamel, waterproofed goods, caulking, paint, wallpaper, gasoline, fire extinguisher foam

SPINACH

See *Goosefoot* Family

Foods • Greek dishes, salads, casseroles, ravioli

STRAWBERRY

See *Rose* Family. Strawberries are known to release histamine from the body; hives may be due to this chemical reaction.

SUGAR

Sugar is not usually considered an allergen; however, the different types are listed here:

Cane • the protein is refined out as the process goes from molasses to brown sugar to cane sugar.

Beet • sucrose, powdered sugar (frequently contains cornstarch)

Maple • tapped from maple trees; usually mixed with cane or corn sugar for commercial preparations.

Sorghum • usually sold in syrup form

Honey • light white sage, orange blossoms, clover blossoms, buckwheat flowers, goldenrod, aster, or honeydew pollen can be part of the honey.

SULFIDES

Courtesy of Scripps Clinic and Research Foundation

Sulfites, bisulfites and metabisulfites are all dry chemical forms of the gas sulfur dioxide, which has been used in food preparation for many centuries. We will refer to all of these compounds as sulfites.

The ancient Egyptians and Romans used the fumes of burning sulfur as a sanitizing agent in wine making, and this practice continues in the modern wine industry. The modern food industry utilizes sulfites in three (3) forms: it is applied as a gas, a solution and a dry powder. The chemicals may be added as preservatives or as sanitizing agents. Most often sulfites are used to prevent discoloration, browning and to crisp (freshen) food during preparation, storage, and distribution.

Information on the commercial use of sulfites is incomplete. The chemicals are found in a wide variety of foods and beverages, however their use is somewhat unpredictable. Sulfites may or may not be listed as an ingredient in prepared foods or drinks. The following list of foods/drinks are likely to contain sulfites.

Salads (including all ingredients in salad bars), potato salad, cole slaw, fruit salad.
Fresh and dried fruits and vegetables ★ (particularly apricots and grapes)
Potatoes - chips, fries, salads, any dehydrated form
Prepared vegetables for salads (in cellophane packages)
Avocados, guacamole, avocado dip (particularly restaurant/commercially prepared)
Shrimp and other seafoods ★
Cider and wine vinegars (rice vinegar is ok), pickled vegetables
Wine, all types
Beer, some types, and other fermented beverages
Processed, preserved, "ready to eat" foods and beverages (in minimal amounts)

★ Peeling or washing these items thoroughly before eating may remove some sulfite.

If you are eating in a restaurant, ask the manager if preservatives, fresheners, crispers, or sulfite solutions/sprays are added to their foods. Remember that although the restaurant may not add sulfites, many commercially prepared products, especially lettuce, potatoes (in any peeled form) and other fresh vegetables purchased by the restaurant may have the substances added.

SWEET GUM

Liquidamber or sweet gum tree (*Altingiaceae*) pollinates in the spring.

SYCAMORE

Sycamore trees (*Platanaceae*) are common pollen but not of major importance to allergy.

TAPIOCA

Derived from the roots of the cassava or manioc tree

Foods • manioc meal, manioc potatoes and bread; sold in pearled, granulated and flaked form as a flour; cassava starch used in yeast cakes and laundry starch; used as thickening agent for pies and other desserts.

TOBACCO

Few people are actually allergic to tobacco. They are irritated by the smoke, aroma or the paper that cigarettes are rolled in. Anyone recently at a gathering of people smoking will have smoke imbedded on his or her clothing, skin, or hair. Smoking in the home while the allergic person is not present is not advisable since smoke can be imbedded in the furnishings, walls, etc.

TOMATO

See *Nightshade* Family

Foods • catsup, chili sauce, salads, salad dressing, sauces and stews

TRAGACANTH GUM

See Vegetable Gums

TUNA

See fish

VEGETABLE GUMS

Include arabic (acacia), karaya (Indian), tragacanth, quince seed, locust bean (carobseed), Irish Moss (carrageenan), chicle, algin, agar, bassora, gelatin, ghatti, gum guar, mesquite, and pectin.It is very difficult to determine what things include vegetable gums because usage changes. If allergic reactions occur after eating or usage of the following, gums should be considered a possible source:

Food

Beverages • chocolate-flavored drinks, evaporated milk, wine (used to clarify), frozen fruit drinks, soft drinks (foam stabilizer), hot and cold drinks (thickener);

Desserts • chocolate products, syrups in frozen products, pastry, cake icing, ice cream (all forms), toppings, whipped cream, meringue, jelly beans and gumdrops, center of soft candy, puddings, baked products, fruit jelly, preserves, jam, gelatins, marshmallows, pie fillings, filled cookies or wafers;

Main Dishes • cheese spreads, processed swiss and cheddar cheese, cream cheese, white sauce, gravies, prepared flour mixes, salad dressings, meat (binder), mustard and other condiments, commercial potato salad, diabetic foods, soybean liquid products

Medical • laxatives, in medications as a filler or emulsifier, intravenous fluid, denture adhesive, powders, tooth powders, mineral oils, lozenges

Other Sources • chewing gum, wave-setting preparations, face powder, rouge, adhesives, sizing materials, printing industry and paper industry, hair dressing, toothpaste, permanent wave sets, mouthwash, shaving lotions, cigar wrappers, stamps, stickers, gummed paper

WALNUTS

See Nuts

Walnut Family (*Juglandaceae*) includes hickories; walnut tree pollen is significant in California and Oregon.

WHEAT

Foods

Beverages • grain drinks such as gin and whiskey; ale, malted milk, prepared milk foods and milk supplements;

Breads • commercially prepared muffins, waffles, biscuits, yeast cakes, rolls, breads, doughnuts, pastries; Flours: buckwheat, corn, graham, lima bean, rye;

Desserts • commercially prepared sherbet and ice cream; commercially prepared cookies, puddings, cakes, pastries, candies, chocolate (except bitter chocolate);

Main Dishes • dumplings, noodles, spaghetti, macaroni, ravioli, soup rings and alphabets, bouillon cakes, yeast cakes, mayonnaise, catsup, salad dressings and gravies, prepared sausages, weiners, luncheon meats, hamburger, bologna, liverwurst

WINE

See Alcoholic Beverages

WILLOW

Poplars and willows (*Salicaceae*) are quite antigenic; however, only the poplar is wind-dispersed

WOOL

Sources • insulation, clothing, carpets, packing, mixed with dog hair to make Chinese rugs

YEASTS

Most common for allergy are *Cryptacoccus*, *Rhodotorula*; Fungi (mold) found in nocturnal, wet weather, during rain and where fruit crops are grown; in the home environment yeasts grow in fluid reservoirs (refrigerator overflows, humidifiers, vaporizers).

Food • Baker's yeast belongs to the *Zygomycetes* Family and *Sacchomyces* genus and *Cervevisae* species, found in baking products

✦ FOR FURTHER INFORMATION

The following list of addresses will assist you in obtaining further information about allergies. Some of the following companies have responded to our request for a description of their services.

ORGANIZATIONS

Allergy Information Association
Room 7
25 Poynter Drive, Suite 7
Weston, Ontario M9RIK8
Canada
(416) 244-9312

Purpose • A.I.A. is a non-profit organization that dispenses allergy information to the general public and to professionals working in related fields. They publish a quarterly newsletter with a circulation of over 4,000. The booklet contains articles helpful to those with allergies. One feature of the newsletter is a review of new books on the market pertaining to allergy.

The Allergy Information Association:

- ✔ enables allergic individuals to increase control over allergy symptoms and improve their health;

- ✔ has joined with the Canadian Society of Allergists and Clinical Immunologists to provide patient education;

- ✔ brings to the attention of manufacturers and government the need for special products and meaningful ingredient listings.

The Allergy Information Association offers practical advice through membership in our association ($20 per annum). Members initially receive a new members' information kit and subscription to A.I.A.'s newsletter—Allergy Quarterly. A.I.A. publishes a series of Information Letters covering many aspects of allergic disease. (Individually priced.) Available are two cookbooks - "Diets Unlimited for Limited Diets" and "Foods for Festive Occasions", developed by members, tested by dietitians, and published by Methuen. ($14.95 each)

Allergy Observer
116 West 32nd Street
New York, New York 10001

(Newsletter)

American Academy of Allergy and Immunology
611 East Wells Street
Milwaukee, WI 53202
(414) 272-6071

Purpose • to advance the knowledge and practice of allergy and immunology through discussion at meetings; to foster the education of both students and the public; to promote and stimulate allergy and immunology research and study and to encourage the unity of and cooperation among those engaged in the field of allergy and immunology.

American Allergy Association

P.O. Box 7273
Menlo Park, California 94026-7273
(415) 322-1663

American Allergy Association publishes an annual handbook, "Living with Allergies," that provides information on allergies to foods, pollens, danders, molds, insects. There are health alerts, book reviews, recipes, questions/answers.

AAA Reports is a series of in-depth articles, providing a closer look at particular allergy problems. Also available are recipes for various allergen-free diets.

Please enclose a stamped, self-addressed long envelope when writing.

American Lung Association

1740 Broadway
New York, NY 10019
(212) 315-8700

Every major city has a branch of the American Lung. Contact the Association for the one nearest you. The Association offers many free booklets including: "Air Pollution in Your Home?" "Home Indoor Air Quality Checklist," "Formaldehyde Fact Sheet," booklets about smoking, and many others.

Asthma & Allergy Foundation of America (AAFA)

1717 Mass Ave. NW, Suite 305
Washington, DC 20036
(202) 265-0265

Purpose • to collect and disseminate information to the public on new research results and basic facts about the causes and treatment of allergic disease; to produce and distribute pamphlets and bulletins; to answer inquiries from the public and from science writers; to arrange for exhibits and professional speakers at public meetings; and to support research in allergy and the training of future allergists through post-doctoral and clinical fellowship.

AAFA published "The Allergy Encyclopedia," (out of print but available at libraries) and a bi-monthly newspaper, the "Advance."

Asthma Care Association of America

P. O. Box 568
Ossining, NY 10362
(914) 762-2110 or 1-800-822-2762 for information

Purpose • Nonprofit corporation dedicated to financially supporting the care, treatment, and rehabilitation of persons with asthma and other allergies; supports research and publishes the Journal of Asthma; makes medical referrals.

Environmental Hazards Management Institute (EHMI)

10 Newmarket Rd., P.O. Box 932
Durham, N.H. 03824
(603) 868-1496

The EHMI offers a Household Hazardous Waste Wheel, a door reference listing the potential hazards of chemical products, and offers nontoxic alternatives.

Environmental Health Watch (EHW)

4115 Bridge Ave.,
Cleveland, Ohio 44113
(216) 961-4646

Purpose • to educate and assist families concerned about the health effects of asbestos, lead, formaldehyde, pesticides, and other materials and products found in the home.

Housing Resource Center (HRC)

1820 W. 48th St
Cleveland, Ohio 44102
(216) 281-4663

Purpose • provides consumers and professionals with practical home-maintenance, repair, and improvement information.

They have a hotline and publish a monthly newsletter, "Your Home," and a quarterly journal,"House-Mending Resources." They sponsor an annual Blueprint for a Healthy House conference.

National Institute of Allergy & Infectious Diseases
NIH
Bethesda , MD 20205

Purpose • to conduct broadly based research and research training in the causes, characteristics, prevention, control, and treatment of a wide variety of diseases, including those believed attributable to allergies or to other deficiencies or disorders in the responses of the body's immune mechanisms.

PRODUCT INFORMATION

Allergy Accessories
4801 J Street
Sacramento, CA 95819
(916) 731-5480

(*sell informational material*)

Allergy Control Products
96 Danbury Rd.
Ridgefield, CT 06877
1-800-DUST

See Advertisement at the end of the book.
(*sell encasings, filters and other allergy products*)

The Al-R-G Shoppe, Inc.
3411 Johnson Street
Hollywood, Florida 33021-9182
(305) 981-9182

(*Catalog of books approved by consultants*)

ATI (Air Techniques, Inc.)
1717 Whitehead Road.
Baltimore, Md 21207

(*HEPA filter*)

Bio-Tech Systems

P. O. Box 25380
Chicago, Ill 60625
(800) 621-5545

(many products by catalog)

Environtrol Corporation

P. O. Box 31313
St. Louis, Mo 63131

(mattress encasings and other products)

HEALTH SERVICES CONSULTANTS

2670 Del Mar Heights Road,
Del Mar, California 92014
(619) 259-6146

*(Writes, Publishes and Markets
Health Education Literature and Training Materials)*

Hi Tech Filter Corp. of America

80 Myrtle St.
No. Quincy, MA 02171
(800) 448-3249

(mechanical filters)

Intertherm Baseboard Heater
Intertherm, Inc.

10820 Sunset Office Drive
St. Louis, MO 63127

(baseboard heaters)

Tectronic Products Company, Inc.

6743 Kinne Street
Post Office Box 157
East Syracuse, New York 13057

(electronic air cleaner, dehumidification equipment)

COSMETICS

Almay Hypo-Allergenic Cosmetics
Schieffelen & Company
625 Madison Avenue
New York, NY 10022
(212) 527-4715

Ar-Ex Cosmetics, Ltd.
233 E Erie, Suite 500
Chicago, IL 60611

Clinique Laboratories, Inc.
Allergy Tested Cosmetics
C.B. 8
Melville, New York 11747

Dermatological Products of Texas, Inc.
P. O. Box 1659
San Antonio, Texas 78296

Neutrogena Dermatologics
Division of **Neutrogena Corp**
Mitchell S. Wortzman, Ph.D.
P. O. Box 45036
Los Angeles, CA 90045

PHARMACEUTICALS MARKETING
ALLERGY PRODUCTS

(*Request patient education literature*)

Abbott Laboratories
Pharmaceutical Products Division
North Chicago, Il 60084

    (*booklets*)

Fisons Corporation
c/o Marketing Department
Pharmaceutical Division
Two Preston Court
Bedford, MA 01730

    Patient Education Literature
    (*Available in English or Spanish*)
    "Your Asthma Answer Book"
    "The Allergy Fact Book...about allergic rhinitis"
    "Allergic Eye Disorders"

Hollister-Stier
Miles Laboratories
400 Morgan Lane
West Haven, CT 06516

    (*booklets on pollens and molds,
    allergy extracts and products*)

Pharmacia Diagnostics
Division of Pharmacia, Inc
800 Centennial Avenue
Piscataway, N.J. 08854

    Patient Education Literature
    "If You Have An Allergy"
    "You and Your Allergy"
    "Timeless Mysteries of Food Allergy"

Ross Laboratories
Division Abbott Laboratories
Columbus, OH 43216

Patient Education Literature

G922 "Your Child and Food Sensitivity"
G970 "Your Milk-Sensitive Infant's First Year"
G714 "Cooking With Isomil"
G333 "Feeding Your Baby a Soy Protein Formula" (English)
G350 "Feeding Your Baby a Soy Protein Formula" (Spanish)
G605 "Allergy Facts Poster"
G135 "Airborne Allergens Poster"
G611 "Understanding Allergy"
G638 "Your First Visit to the Allergist"
(*counseling pad*)

G653 "What Causes Allergy?" (*counseling pad*)
G654 "Allergic Rhinitis" (*counseling pad*)
G655 "Allergy Tests" (*counseling pad*)
G351 "Allergy Proofing Your Home" (*counseling pad*)

Schering Corporation
Galloping Hill Road
Kenilworth, NJ 07033

Searle Pharmaceuticals Inc.
Box 5110
Chicago, IL 60077

Patient education information:
"Active with Asthma"
by:
C. Warren Bierman M.D.
Gail G. Shapiro M.D.
William E. Pierson M.D.

◆ APPENDIX

POLLENS

We were granted permission by Miles Laboratory to print the following book published by Hollister-Stier Laboratories, "Pollen Guide For Allergy," by Ray Nelson. It is a mini botany course that provides an excellent foundation for understanding pollen bearing plants that result in hay fever.

POLLEN GUIDE FOR ALLERGY

By RAY NELSON *

It has been said that no man is an island and today with our heightened environmental awareness, we have a much broader concept of mankind's place on earth.

On every continent there are geographic regions delineated by natural components: mountains, rivers, and seacoasts. Geologic and climatic phenomena have created numerous regions with characteristic soils, water, and weather which become the natural habitat of seemingly infinite plant variety and adaptation. These regions attract man, too; especially in this age and on this continent, individuals migrate to their preferred climate to the region where they feel at home. So mankind imposes himself into areas already occupied by the indigenous plant life, and intermingles with a complex ecosystem.

Man is by no means ever satisfied with his environment, and out of his own needs and desires he changes it through agriculture and the building of cities. Competition for survival between plants and man is a never-ending struggle. Man also has desires and needs for travel; out of the machine age has come a system of transportation and mobility which has made him a virtual nomad, moving not only within but between continents in incredibly short time, and exposing himself to diverse plant life as never before.

In any investigation of hay fever (pollinosis), it is necessary to look at geography first, to assess the distribution of human populations as well as plant populations. Obviously where there are few people, there is little pollinosis, nor can there be pollinosis (regardless of population size) where there are no plants which produce allergenic pollen.

* Botanist, Hollister-Stier Laboratories

Plants, too, live not only in biogeographic and climatic regions, but also in smaller communities with rather well defined parameters and components. On a global scale, the major climatic regions, and consequently the plant communities, vary with latitude and altitude.

In general, temperatures are inversely proportionate to degrees in latitude. We acknowledge this principle when we select our garden and landscape plants to suit our local climate; we should always consider temperatures when assessing the hay fever flora of any region. In the arctic, and at high altitudes, the average maximum temperatures are so low that the few plants which exist are sparse in number and dwarf in size, seldom exceeding several inches in height. Summers are so short that many arctic and alpine plants, even grasses and dwarf willows, reproduce vegetatively (asexually), avoiding the energy expense and risk of producing pollen and setting seed. And in the subartic, the predominant plants are the evergreen conifers which shed copious amounts of hypoallergenic pollen.

At the other extreme, many parts of the tropics are so humid that anemophilous (wind-borne) pollen is rare. Pollen is hygroscopic (absorbs atmospheric water vapor), and in the humid tropics pollen absorbs too much moisture therefore it is too heavy for wind transport. Another peculiarity of the tropics and subtropics is the great proliferation of numbers of species with a relative decline in numbers of individuals per species. Survival of the species depends on many specific pollinators, such as bats, birds, and insects — the pollen being unavailable to any but the "right" pollinator.

Therefore, hay fever plants and consequently hay fever are limited to the temperate regions, each with its own peculiar biogeographic regions, and plant communities, yet sharing much in common on the continental basis. (Southern California, the Gulf Coast, and especially southern Florida have virtually a subtropic flora and some peculiar hay fever problems which are not fully understood at this time.)

Pollen is so common that its true nature is often unrecognized. First, pollen is produced only by seed-bearing plants, viz., the conifers and flowering plants. Algae, fungi, mosses, and ferns do not produce pollen. The pollen grain is "descended" from the fern spore in a sense, and is very similar in appearance in some species of flowering plants, but it is quite different from a spore in function. The pollen grain is analogous to a spermatozoon in that like a male gamete, it is a haploid unit. When pollination occurs, a double fertilization follows, with the development of an embryonic plant and a nutritive tissue (endosperm). Were pollen only a sperm, its size might be so ˙reduced as to be insignificant as an agent or respiratory allergy.

Normally only anemophilous pollen can cause hay fever. Thommen's five postulates give us a concise profile of a hay fever plant:

1 ● The plant must be seed-bearing (spermatophyte); only seed-bearing plants produce pollen.

2 ● The plant must have wide distribution, or the plant must be close to the human environment.

3 ● The plant must produce large quantities of pollen.

4 ● The pollen must be light enough to be airborne, between 15 and 50 microns diameter.

6 ● The pollen must be allergenic.

Any species which fits all five postulates may be considered a primary or index species. If the profile is incomplete, the species in question might still be a problem for some people, but its overall significance is greatly reduced.

Because the pollen grain is a functional unit of transfer of genetic material, it has been of much interest to botanists. Pollen ecologists, who are concerned with the dispersal of pollen, have given us another profile which can be used to identify an anemophilous plant. It is a microscopic examination of the flower(s), and anyone can decide for himself, with accuracy, if wind is the normal pollen vector.

POLLEN GUIDE FOR ALLERGY *CONTINUED* —

So what is an anemophilous plant?

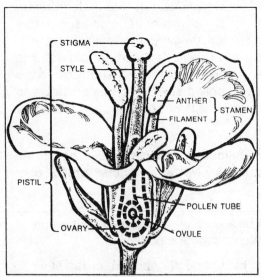

FLOWER CROSS SECTION shows a cluster of stamens, each with apollen-gilled anther at its tip, surrounding a central pistil with a sticky stigma at the tip and an ovary in the base. One pollen grain adhering to the stigma ahs grown a long tube reaching the ovary.

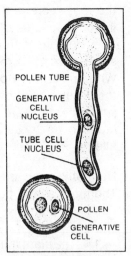

GRAIN OF POLLEN.

If a free pollen grain comes in contact with a stigma, the tube cell becomes involved with the growth of the pollen tube toward the ovary and the generative cell then travels down the tube to fertilize the ovule.

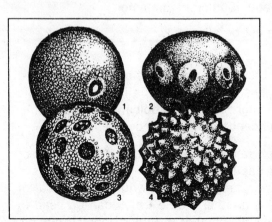

2. *JUGLANS NIGRA, side view dorsal side uppermost,* 34 μ *in diameter.*

3. *SALSOLA PESTIFER, 27.5 μ in diameter.*

4. *AMBROSIA TRIFIDA, 17.7 μ in diameter.*

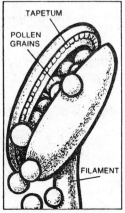

ANTHER, which splits at maturity allowing the loose pollen in its cavities to disperse.

So what is an anemophilous plant?

1 ● The flowers are unisexual (imperfect), either pollen producers or pollen receptors, but not both.

2 ● The flowers are exposed to the wind, either before the leaves appear, or outside the leaf-mass.

3 ● The petals and sepals, which make most flowers attractive to humans as well as to insects, are reduced in size to insignificance or are absent altogether. Anemophilous flowers are unattractive.

4 ● The anther (pollen-producing structures) and stigmas (pollen receptors) are exposed and conspicuous.

5 ● Attractants like odors, nectars, brilliant colors are absent.

6 ● The pollen grains are small (25 to 50 microns diameter), smooth (surface ornaments reduced or absent) and dry (not sticky with fats, pigments, and waxes).

7 ● Mechanisms for arresting pollen release are frequently present, so that pollen is released only by the violent shaking action of the wind (otherwise the pollen would fall to the ground in calm air, and not achieve its function).

With Thommen's postulates and the profile of anemophily in mind, one can go anywhere and indicate the potential hay fever plants.* To determine whether a pollen is allergenic however, the pollen or its extract must be clinically tested in known sensitive patients to that specific pollen, or tested in vitro in the laboratory by sophisticated testing procedures. Some plants, like the majority of the conifers (except *Juniperus* and *Cupressus*) and sweet gum (*Liquidambar*), although prodigious in pollen production, seem to be relatively hypoallergenic.

---

* Gymnosperms represent anemophily; i.e., throughout geologic time they have been wind pollinated. Angiosperms represent primary entomophily; i.e., in geologic time they originated as insect-pollinated plants, and subsequently some angiosperm groups became anemophilous. The allergens may be vestiges of a biochemical mechanism against self-fertilization in entomophilous plants.

The identification and mapping of hay fever flora is a highly advanced stage in the United States. Of the thousands or more species of anemophilous plants in North America, the pollens of only some three hundred species are commonly extracted for clinical testing, and perhaps only 100 species continent-wide are primary offenders.

Many entomophilous (insect vector) plants have strong pollen antigens, some of which may be actual irritants, but these are of very minor significance because the grains are not inhaled. Thus among children playing in a dandelion patch, the dandelion pollen might cause pollinosis, but not in the general population. In a few species, e.g. linden (*Tilia*), insects are the usual pollen vectors, and the plant fits neither Thommen's postulates nor the profile of anemophily at the onset of anthesis (opening of the flower); however, near the end of the pollination period the pollen, still in excess of actual needs to assure fertilization, dries out and becomes airborne. Although it may no longer be viable, the allergens may still be potent and the pollen may cause hay fever. Such species are few and may include *Eucalyptus*, willows (*Salix*), some maples (*Acer*), *Acacia*, and some other trees.

Plants are always found in plant communities, natural aggregations of organisms which have nutual relationships with one another and with the physical environment. Some plant communities may be altered, as in the North Dakota wheat fields where all organisms except wheat are suppressed; yet as soon as the farmers' vigilance wanes, the "weeds" are ready to return and make a mixed community again. With each community there is competition for light, space, mineral nutrients, and water. Under ideal circumstances the plants will grow to the limits of their environment but neither more nor less. On the deserts, where water is the limiting factor, individual plants are widely spaced yet filling as much of the space as water supply permits. A well watered meadow might have hundreds of individual plants per square meter, being limited only by their ability to have leaves exposed to the sun.

Fires, floods, erosion, and human industry all prepare barren soil for which the adapted species compete, in one form succeeding another until a stable, integrated community is achieved—the climax. At this point the dominant vegetation is the tallest that the environment will support, the dominant plants having outgrown everything else. hay fever plants are found in all stages of this competitive succession and their broad classification as weeds, grasses, and trees reflects their importance in the environment better than any taxonomic scheme.

Start with a barren piece of land, such as a flooded riverbank, a burned-over woodland, a plowed field, or a disked vacant lot in Toronto. The first plants which appear are the weeds, vigorous and invasive, which seemingly thrive on the poorest soil and grow luxuriantly under the most adverse conditions. The weeds, however, are short-lived, and cannot tolerate competition. If left undisturbed, they will die out in natural progression as the grasses and other perennials take over, surviving by their deep roots and ability to endure the changing seasons. Utimately the grasses and perennial weeds will be shaded to death by shrubs, if there is sufficient water to support them, and the shrubs are overcome by trees if there is sufficient water to support them. In hay fever literature certain desert species are called weeds for want of a better term, e.g., *Franseria dumosa, DESERT RAGWEED*, but in the native environment they are small shrubs, the largest plant forms that the environment will support. Using the concept of plant succession with limiting factors, certain regional patterns can be seen: the warm desert of the southwestern U.S., the cold deserts of the intermountain northwestern U.S., the deciduous forest of southeastern Canada and northeastern U.S., the coastal forest of the Pacific provinces and states, the Rocky Mountain provinces and states with their many vegetational zones according to altitude, and the prairie grasslands of southcentral Canada and central U.S. where the only native trees are found along watercourses. The plant communities are adapted to their geographic regions, and those regions are characterized by their indigenous plant species.

Mankind has a way of disturbing the natural order of life unlike any other factor. The practice of clearing land for man's use continues yearly, perhaps with increasing acceleration, creating a thriving, large, bothersome, unnatural weed population. Mixed ranges of grass are replaced by a few introduced species. City streets are lined with introduced trees. In every part of our environment, we see the human influence abetting the proliferation of hay fever plants — fostering human misery.

Taxonomy (from Greek, an orderly naming system) tends to discourage — if not intimidate-physicians from personal investigation of botanic literature. Once every decade botanists hold an international congress, a division of which governs the naming of plants. Legal codes change with additions, deletions, and revisions to reflect the changes in society. Likewise, rules of plant nomenclature change to reflect increasing global understanding of plant relationships and distribution. Just as laws can be traced back through antiquity, so *technical* names of plants can be traced through any changes that might have been made. Common names, on the other hand, are uncontrolled and highly variable, and very often conflicting. Nobody is advocating the abolition of common names, for they have a very important place; but the physician who develops some awareness of the technical names (the latinized binominal) will understand more about plant affinities.

In the diagnosis and treatment of pollinosis, the physician is not really concerned with the plant name, but with the air-borne pollen grains as contaminating foreign particles of specific allergens and combinations of allergens. Any special concern over nomenclature and identification is merely to assure that the physician is using pollen extracts representative of the pollen antigens in the environment of his patients. We should keep in mind that a single plant rarely causes pollinosis because pollinosis is an effect of populations of plants on populations of humans, both of which inhabit the same or close by geographic areas. As a community health problem, the physician must necessarily be concerned with his own regional flora.

Too few physicians make their own personal analyses of their regional hay fever floras because of the time, equipment and knowledge required. Many cities, counties, and states make surveys of their floras and aerial samples for determination of pollen counts. Over the years this body of data has grown so that now there is a relatively complete overview of both regional and continental allergy. That data has been compiled, reviewed, and condensed to present each physician with a *concise* picture of the *primary* hay fever plants within his general region. This is the basis for regional diagnostic sets. The physician's regionalized set is not complete in that every allergic pollen extract is not included. It is a practical and valuable application of Thommen's postulates, emphasizing those species which are most common and present the majority of hay fever problems.

The delineation of regional allergy is not easy. No two communities are identical, yet many adjacent regions share common hay fever floras. Certain seasonal winds from the deserts in southeastern California bring pollen hundreds of miles to the Los Angeles basin, causing serious allergy problems for people who are quite removed from the offending plants. In mountainous regions, the winds can transport pollen from the higher elevations to communities in the foothills and valleys. In defining hay fever regions, prevailing winds, seasonal winds and elevation are decisive factors for the inclusion (or exclusion) of primary offending species.

The physician is not limited to the species included in his regional set, and he should add supplemental species where he feels they are important in his community. It would be unwise to delete species since they were included because of their primary significance. Sometimes it is necessary to supplement a set with diagnostic extracts of pollen indigenous to other regions to test and treat patients who have moved their residence but continue to travel among different botanical regions.

The diagnosis and treatment of pollinosis begins with pure, fresh, accurately identified pollen. The raw pollen is collected directly from the plant wherever the pollen is:

1 ● most representative of the continental population of each species;

2 ● very abundant, therefore most economical to collect;

3 ● least likely to be contaminated by other environmental pollutants...

The following charts have been furnished by Hollister-Stier for future reference on various areas of the country.

MAJOR BOTANICAL AREAS

The United States and Canada are divided into twenty-one (21) regions. The regions are generally composed of contiguous areas having similar climatic and geographical features. State and Province boundaries may be used for easy identification whenever possible, but other boundaries may be identified by counties within states, or major geographical features.

Region I

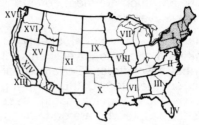

North Atlantic U.S.A.

STATES:

Connecticut	Maine
Massachusetts	New Hampshire
New Jersey	New York
Pennsylvania	Rhode Island
Vermont	

VEGETATION:

Trees—Appalachian oak forest and northern hardwood forest (beech, birch, hemlock, and maple).

Grasses—Several genera, naturalized and/or cultivated for hay and lawns, although inconspicuous, are very abundant and significant in hayfever.

Weeds—Although relatively few species of weeds are important, their widespread abundance and heavy pollination over a long season make them important hayfever plants.

INDEX TREES: (Pollinating Season—Late Winter through Spring)

BOX ELDER/MAPLE (*Acer spp.*)
BIRCH (*Betula spp.*)
OAK (*Quercus spp.*)
HICKORY (*Carya ovata*)
ASH (*Fraxinus americana*)
PINE (*Pinus strobus*)
SYCAMORE (*Platanus occidentalis*)
COTTONWOOD/POPLAR (*Populus deltoides*)
ELM (*Ulmus americana*)

INDEX GRASSES: (Pollinating Season—Spring through Early Summer)

  REDTOP (*Agrostis alba*)
  ORCHARD (*Dactylis glomerata*)
  FESCUE (*Festuca elatior*)
  TIMOTHY (*Phleum pratense*)
  BLUEGRASS/JUNEGRASS (*Poa spp.*)

INDEX WEEDS: (Pollinating Season—Summer through Early Fall)

  LAMB'S QUARTERS (*Chenopodium album*)
  RAGWEED, GIANT & SHORT (*Ambrosia spp.*)
  COCKLEBUR (*Xanthium strumarium*)
  PLANTAIN (*Plantago lanceolata*)
  DOCK/SORREL (*Rumex spp.*)

Region II

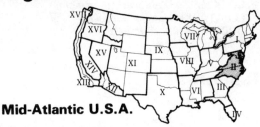

Mid-Atlantic U.S.A.

STATES:

Delaware	District of Columbia
Maryland	North Carolina
Virginia	

VEGETATION:

Trees—Appalachian oak forest and oak-hickory-pine forest.

Grasses—Several genera, naturalized and/or cultivated for hay and lawns, although inconspicuous, are very abundant and significant in hayfever.

Weeds—Although relatively few species of weeds are important, their widespread abundance and heavy pollination over a long season make them important hayfever plants.

INDEX TREES: (Pollinating Season—Late Winter through Spring)

  BOX ELDER/MAPLE (*Acer spp.*)
  BIRCH (*Betula nigra*)
  CEDAR/JUNIPER (*Juniperus virginiana*)
  OAK (*Quercus spp.*)
  HICKORY/PECAN (*Carya spp.*)
  WALNUT (*Juglans nigra*)
  MULBERRY (*Morus spp.*)
  ASH (*Fraxinus americana*)
  COTTONWOOD/POPLAR (*Populus deltoides*)
  HACKBERRY (*Celtis occidentalis*)
  ELM (*Ulmus americana*)

INDEX GRASSES: (Pollinating Season—Spring through Early Summer)
   REDTOP (*Agrostis alba*)
   VERNALGRASS (*Anthoxanthum sp.*)
   BERMUDAGRASS (*Cynodon dactylon*)
   ORCHARDGRASS (*Dactylis glomerata*)
   RYEGRASS (*Elymus & lolium spp.*)
   TIMOTHY (*Phleum pratense*)
   BLUEGRASS/JUNEGRASS (*Poa spp.*)
   JOHNSONGRASS (*Sorghum halepense*)

INDEX WEEDS: (Pollinating Season—Summer through Early Fall)
   PIGWEED (*Amaranthus retroflexus*)
   LAMB'S QUARTERS (*Chenopodium album*)
   MEXICAN FIREBUSH (*Kochia scoparia*)
   RAGWEED, GIANT & SHORT (*Ambrosia spp.*)
   COCKLEBUR (*Xanthium strumarium*)
   PLANTAIN (*Plantago lanceolata*)
   DOCK/SORREL (*Rumex spp.*)

Region III

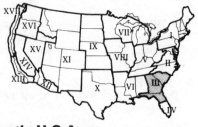

South Atlantic U.S.A.

STATES:
   Florida, Northern, (above Orlando)
   Georgia   South Carolina

VEGETATION:
   Trees—Oak-hickory-pine forest and southern mixed forest (beech, oak, pine).

   Grasses—Several genera, naturalized and/or cultivated for hay and lawns, although inconspicuous, are very abundant and significant in hayfever.

   Weeds—Although relatively few species of weeds are important, their widespread abundance and heavy pollination over a long season make them important hayfever plants.

INDEX TREES: (Pollinating Season—Late Winter through Spring)
BOX ELDER/MAPLE (*Acer spp.*)
BIRCH (*Betula nigra*)
CEDAR/JUNIPER (*Juniperus virginiana*)
OAK (*Quercus spp.*)
HICKORY/PECAN (*Carya spp.*)
WALNUT (*Juglans nigra*)
MESQUITE (*Prosopis juliflora*)
MULBERRY (*Morus spp.*)
ASH (*Fraxinus americana*)
COTTONWOOD/POPLAR (*Populus deltoides*)
HACKBERRY (*Celtis occidentalis*)
ELM (*Ulmus americana*)

INDEX GRASSES: (Pollinating Season—Spring through Early Summer)
REDTOP (*Agrostis alba*)
VERNALGRASS (*Anthoxanthum sp.*)
BERMUDAGRASS (*Cynodon dactylon*)
ORCHARDGRASS (*Dactylis glomerata*)
RYEGRASS (*Elymus & Lolium spp.*)
FESCUE (*Festuca elatior*)
TIMOTHY (*Phleum pratense*)
BLUEGRASS/JUNEGRASS (*Poa spp.*)
JOHNSONGRASS (*Sorghum halepense*)

INDEX WEEDS: (Pollinating Season—Summer through Early Fall)
LAMB'S QUARTERS (*Chenopodium album*)
RAGWEED, GIANT & SHORT (*Ambrosia spp.*)
SAGEBRUSH (*Artemisia spp.*)
COCKLEBUR (*Xanthium strumarium*)
PLANTAIN (*Plantago lanceolata*)
DOCK/SORREL (*Rumex spp.*)

Region IV

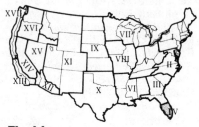

Subtropic Florida

STATES:
Florida, Southern (Below Orlando)

VEGETATION:

Trees—Southern mixed forest, palmetto prairie, and everglades.

Grasses—Several genera, naturalized and/or cultivated for hay and lawns, although inconspicuous, are very abundant and significant in hayfever.

Weeds—Although relatively few species of weeds are important, their widespread abundance and heavy pollination over a long season make them important hayfever plants.

INDEX TREES: (Pollinating Season—Winter through Spring)
BOX ELDER (*Acer negundo*)
CEDAR/JUNIPER (*Juniperus virginiana*)
OAK (*Quercus spp.*)
PECAN (*Carya pecan*)
PRIVET (*Ligustrum lucidum*)
PALM (*Cocos plumosa*)
AUSTRALIAN PINE (BEEFWOOD) (*Casuarina equisetifolia*)
SYCAMORE (*Platanus occidentalis*)
COTTONWOOD/POPLAR (*Populus deltoides*)
ELM (*Ulmus americana*)
BRAZILIAN PEPPERTREE (FLORIDA HOLLY) (*Schinus terebinthifolius*)
BAYBERRY (WAX MYRTLE) (*Myrica spp.*)
MELALEUCA (*Melaleuca sp.*)

INDEX GRASSES: (Pollinating Season—Spring through Early Summer)
REDTOP (*Agrostis alba*)
BERMUDAGRASS (*Cynodon dactylon*)
SALTGRASS (*Distichlis sp.*)
BAHIAGRASS (*Paspalum notatum*)
CANARYGRASS (*Phalaris minor*)
BLUEGRASS/JUNEGRASS (*Poa spp.*)
JOHNSONGRASS (*Sorghum halepense*)

INDEX WEEDS: (Pollinating Season—Summer through Early Fall)
PIGWEED (*Amaranthus spinosus*)
LAMB'S QUARTERS (*Chenopodium album*)
RAGWEED, GIANT & SHORT (*Ambrosia spp.*)
SAGEBRUSH (*Artemisia spp.*)
MARSH ELDER/POVERTY WEED (*Iva spp.*)
DOCK/SORREL (*Rumex spp.*)
PLANTAIN (*Plantago lanceolata*)

Region V

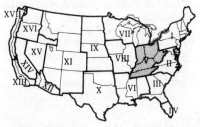

The Greater Ohio Valley

STATES:

Indiana	Kentucky
Ohio	Tennessee
West Virginia	

VEGETATION:

Trees—Mixed forest (beech, maple, oak), beech-maple forest, and oak-hickory forest.

Grasses—Several genera, naturalized and/or cultivated for hay and lawns, although inconspicuous, are very abundant and significant in hayfever.

Weeds—Although relatively few species of weeds are important, their widespread abundance and heavy pollination over a long season make them important hayfever plants.

INDEX TREES: (Pollinating Season—Late Winter through Spring)
- BOX ELDER/MAPLE (*Acer spp.*)
- BIRCH (*Betula nigra*)
- OAK (*Quercus rubra*)
- HICKORY (*Carya ovata*)
- WALNUT (*Juglans nigra*)
- ASH (*Fraxinus americana*)
- SYCAMORE (*Platanus occidentalis*)
- COTTONWOOD/POPLAR (*Populus deltoides*)
- ELM (*Ulmus americana*)

INDEX GRASSES: (Pollinating Season—Spring through Early Summer)
- REDTOP (*Agrostis alba*)
- BERMUDAGRASS (*Cynodon dactylon*)
- ORCHARDGRASS (*Dactylis glomerata*)
- FESCUE (*Festuca elatior*)
- RYEGRASS (*Lolium spp.*)
- TIMOTHY (*Phleum pratense*)
- BLUEGRASS/JUNEGRASS (*Poa spp.*)
- JOHNSONGRASS (*Sorghum halepense*)

INDEX WEEDS: (Pollinating Season—Summer through Early Fall)
- WATERHEMP (*Acnida tamariscina*)
- PIGWEED (*Amaranthus retroflexus*)
- LAMB'S QUARTERS (*Chenopodium album*)
- RAGWEED, GIANT & SHORT (*Ambrosia spp.*)
- SAGEBRUSH (*Artemisia spp.*)
- COCKLEBUR (*Xanthium strumarium*)
- DOCK/SORREL (*Rumex spp.*)
- PLANTAIN (*Plantago lanceolata*)

Region VI

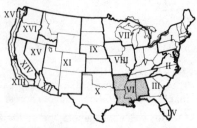

South Central U.S.A.

STATES:

Alabama	Arkansas
Louisiana	Mississippi

VEGETATION:

Trees—Southern flood plain forest, surrounded by oak-hickory-pine forest and oak-hickory forest.

Grasses—Several genera, naturalized and/or cultivated for hay and lawns, although inconspicuous, are very abundant and significant in hayfever.

Weeds—Although relatively few species of weeds are important, their widespread abundance and heavy pollination over a long season make them important hayfever plants.

INDEX TREES: (Pollinating Season—Late Winter through Spring)
- BOX ELDER/MAPLE (*Acer spp.*)
- CEDAR/JUNIPER (*Juniperus virginiana*)
- OAK (*Quercus spp.*)
- HICKORY/PECAN (*Carya spp.*)
- WALNUT (*Juglans nigra*)
- ASH (*Fraxinus americana*)
- SYCAMORE (*Platanus occidentalis*)
- COTTONWOOD/POPLAR (*Populus deltoides*)
- HACKBERRY (*Celtis occidentalis*)
- ELM (*Ulmus americana*)

INDEX GRASSES: (Pollinating Season—Spring through Early Summer)
  REDTOP (*Agrostis alba*)
  BERMUDAGRASS (*Cynodon dactylon*)
  ORCHARDGRASS (*Dactylis glomerata*)
  RYEGRASS (*Lolium spp.*)
  TIMOTHY (*Phleum pratense*)
  BLUEGRASS/JUNEGRASS (*Poa spp.*)
  JOHNSONGRASS (*Sorghum halepense*)

INDEX WEEDS: (Pollinating Season—Summer through Early Fall)
  CARELESSWEED/PIGWEED (*Amaranthus spp.*)
  LAMB'S QUARTERS (*Chenopodium album*)
  RAGWEED, GIANT & SHORT (*Ambrosia spp.*)
  SAGEBRUSH (*Artemisia spp.*)
  MARSH ELDER/POVERTY WEED (*Iva spp.*)
  COCKLEBUR (*Xanthium strumarium*)
  PLANTAIN (*Plantago lanceolata*)
  DOCK/SORREL (*Rumex spp.*)

Region VII

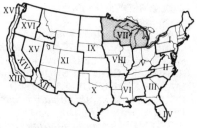

The Northern Midwest

STATES:

Michigan	Minnesota
Wisconsin	

VEGETATION:

Trees—Northern hardwood and Great Lakes pine forests, bluestem prairie and oak savannahs.

Grasses—Several genera, naturalized and/or cultivated for hay and lawns, although inconspicuous, are very abundant and significant in hayfever.

Weeds—Although relatively few species of weeds are important, their widespread abundance and heavy pollination over a long season make them important hayfever plants.

INDEX TREES: (Pollinating Season—Late Winter through Spring)
BOX ELDER/MAPLE (*Acer spp.*)
ALDER (*Alnus incana*)
BIRCH (*Betula spp.*)
OAK (*Quercus rubra*)
HICKORY (*Carya ovata*)
WALNUT (*Juglans nigra*)
ASH (*Fraxinus americana*)
SYCAMORE (*Platanus occidentalis*)
COTTONWOOD/POPLAR (*Populus deltoides*)
ELM (*Ulmus americana*)

INDEX GRASSES: (Pollinating Season—Spring through Early Summer)
REDTOP (*Agrostis alba*)
BROME (*Bromus inermis*)
ORCHARDGRASS (*Dactylis glomerata*)
FESCUE (*Festuca elatior*)
RYEGRASS (*Lolium spp.*)
CANARYGRASS (*Phalaris arundinacea*)
TIMOTHY (*Phleum pratense*)
BLUEGRASS/JUNEGRASS (*Poa spp.*)

INDEX WEEDS: (Pollinating Season—Summer through Early Fall)
WATERHEMP (*Acnida tamariscina*)
LAMB'S QUARTERS (*Chenopodium album*)
RUSSIAN THISTLE (*Salsola kali*)
RAGWEED, GIANT & SHORT (*Ambrosia spp.*)
MARSH ELDER/POVERTY WEED (*Iva spp.*)
COCKLEBUR (*Xanthium strumarium*)
DOCK/SORREL (*Rumex spp.*)
PIGWEED (*Amaranthus retroflexus*)
PLANTAIN (*Plantago lanceolata*)

Region VIII

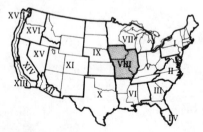

The Central Midwest

STATES:
Illinois   Iowa
Missouri

VEGETATION:

Trees—Mixed bluestem prairie and oak-hickory forest, and relatively large mixed areas.

Grasses—Several genera, naturalized and/or cultivated for hay and lawns, although inconspicuous, are very abundant and significant in hayfever.

Weeds—Although relatively few species of weeds are important, their widespread abundance and heavy pollination over a long season make them important hayfever plants.

INDEX TREES: (Pollinating Season—Late Winter through Spring)

BOX ELDER/MAPLE (*Acer spp.*)
BIRCH (*Betula nigra*)
OAK (*Quercus spp.*)
HICKORY (*Carya ovata*)
WALNUT (*Juglans nigra*)
MULBERRY (*Morus spp.*)
ASH (*Fraxinus americana*)
SYCAMORE (*Platanus occidentalis*)
COTTONWOOD/POPLAR (*Populus deltoides*)
ELM (*Ulmus americana*)

INDEX GRASSES: (Pollinating Season—Spring through Early Summer)

REDTOP (*Agrostis alba*)
BERMUDAGRASS (*Cynodon dactylon*)
ORCHARDGRASS (*Dactylis glomerata*)
RYEGRASS (*Lolium spp.*)
TIMOTHY (*Phleum pratense*)
BLUEGRASS/JUNEGRASS (*Poa spp.*)
JOHNSONGRASS (*Sorghum halepense*)
CORN (*Zea mays*)

INDEX WEEDS: (Pollinating Season—Summer through Early Fall)

PIGWEED (*Amaranthus retroflexus*)
LAMB'S QUARTERS (*Chenopodium album*)
MEXICAN FIREBUSH (*Kochia scoparia*)
RUSSIAN THISTLE (*Salsola kali*)
RAGWEED, GIANT, SHORT & WESTERN
    (*Ambrosia spp.*)
MARSH ELDER/POVERTY WEED (*Iva spp.*)
PLANTAIN (*Plantago lanceolata*)
DOCK/SORREL (*Rumex spp.*)
WATERHEMP (*Acnida tamariscina*)

Region IX

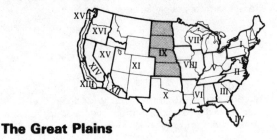

The Great Plains

STATES:

Kansas   Nebraska
North Dakota   South Dakota

VEGETATION:

Trees—Mixed prairies; predominant trees culti-vated.

Grasses—This region is predominantly grassland, but the more important hayfever grasses are cul-tivated for hay or lawns, or are naturalized pests.

Weeds—Although relatively few species of weeds are important, their widespread abundance and heavy pollination over a long season make them important hayfever plants.

INDEX TREES: (Pollinating Season—Late Winter through Spring)
BOX ELDER/MAPLE (*Acer spp.*)
ALDER (*Alnus incana*)
BIRCH (*Betula spp.*)
HAZELNUT (*Corylus americana*)
OAK (*Quercus macrocarpa*)
HICKORY (*Carya ovata*)
WALNUT (*Juglans nigra*)
ASH (*Fraxinus americana*)
COTTONWOOD/POPLAR (*Populus deltoides*)
ELM (*Ulmus americana*)

INDEX GRASSES: (Pollinating Season—Spring through Early Summer)
QUACKGRASS/WHEATGRASS (*Agropyron spp.*)
REDTOP (*Agrostis alba*)
BROME (*Bromus inermis*)
ORCHARDGRASS (*Dactylis glomerata*)
RYEGRASS (*Elymus & Lolium spp.*)
FESCUE (*Festuca elatior*)
TIMOTHY (*Phleum pratense*)
BLUEGRASS/JUNEGRASS (*Poa spp.*)

  WATERHEMP (*Acnida tamariscina*)
  PIGWEED (*Amaranthus retroflexus*)
  LAMB'S QUARTERS (*Chenopodium album*)
  MEXICAN FIREBUSH (*Kochia scoparia*)
  RUSSIAN THISTLE (*Salsola kali*)
  RAGWEED, FALSE, GIANT, SHORT &
    WESTERN (*Ambrosia spp.*)
  SAGEBRUSH (*Artemisia spp.*)
  MARSH ELDER/POVERTY WEED (*Iva spp.*)
  COCKLEBUR (*Xanthium strumarium*)
  PLANTAIN (*Plantago lanceolata*)
  DOCK/SORREL (*Rumex spp.*)

Region X

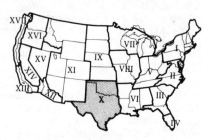

Southwestern Grasslands

STATES:
  Oklahoma   Texas

VEGETATION:
  Trees — Shrub savannah in the west and south, central and northern mixed prairies, and eastern oak-hickory-pine forests.

  Grasses — This region is predominantly grassland, but the more important hayfever grasses are cultivated for hay or lawns, or are naturalized pests.

  Weeds — Although relatively few species of weeds are important, their widespread abundance and heavy pollination over a long season make them important hayfever plants.

INDEX TREES: (Pollinating Season — Late Winter through Spring)
  BOX ELDER (*Acer negundo*)
  CEDAR/JUNIPER (*Juniperus virginiana*)
  OAK (*Quercus virginiana*)
  MESQUITE (*Prosopis juliflora*)
  MULBERRY (*Morus spp.*)
  ASH (*Fraxinus americana*)
  COTTONWOOD/POPLAR (*Populus deltoides*)
  ELM (*Ulmus americana*)

INDEX GRASSES: (Pollinating Season—Spring through Early Summer)

  QUACKGRASS/WHEATGRASS (*Agropyron spp.*)
  REDTOP (*Agrostis alba*)
  BERMUDAGRASS (*Cynodon dactylon*)
  ORCHARDGRASS (*Dactylis glomerata*)
  FESCUE (*Festuca elatior*)
  RYEGRASS (*Lolium spp.*)
  TIMOTHY (*Phleum pratense*)
  BLUEGRASS/JUNEGRASS (*Poa spp.*)
  JOHNSONGRASS (*Sorghum halepense*)

INDEX WEEDS: (Pollinating Season—Summer through Early Fall)

  WATERHEMP (*Acnida tamariscina*)
  CARELESS WEED/PIGWEED (*Amaranthus spp.*)
  SALTBUSH/SCALE (*Atriplex spp.*)
  LAMB'S QUARTERS (*Chenopodium album*)
  MEXICAN FIREBUSH (*Kochia scoparia*)
  RUSSIAN THISTLE (*Salsola kali*)
  RAGWEED, FALSE, GIANT, SHORT &
    WESTERN (*Ambrosia spp.*)
  SAGEBRUSH (*Artemisia spp.*)
  MARSH ELDER/POVERTY WEED (*Iva spp.*)
  COCKELBUR (*Xanthium strumarium*)
  DOCK/SORREL (*Rumex spp.*)
  PLANTAIN (*Plantago lanceolata*)

Region XI

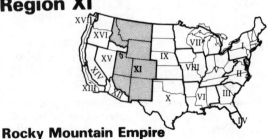

Rocky Mountain Empire

STATES:

  Arizona (Mountainous) Colorado
  Idaho (Mountainous)   Montana
  New Mexico   Utah
  Wyoming

VEGETATION:

Trees—Mixed prairies and steppes to pinyon-juniper woodlands and mixed conifer forests, from lower elevation and latitude to higher.

Grasses—Several genera, naturalized and/or cultivated for hay and lawns, although inconspicuous, are very abundant and significant in hay-fever.

Weeds—Although relatively few species of weeds are important, their widespread abundance and heavy pollination over a long season make them important hayfever plants.

INDEX TREES: (Pollinating Season—Late Winter through Spring)
BOX ELDER (*Acer negundo*)
ALDER (*Alnus incana*)
BIRCH (*Betula fontinalis*)
CEDAR/JUNIPER (*Juniperus scopulorum*)
OAK (*Quercus gambelii*)
ASH (*Fraxinus americana*)
PINE (*Pinus spp.*)
COTTONWOOD/POPLAR (*Populus deltoides*)
    (*sargentii*)
ELM (*Ulmus spp.*)

INDEX GRASSES: (Pollinating Season—Spring through Early Summer)
QUACKGRASS/WHEATGRASS (*Agropyron spp.*)
REDTOP (*Agrostis alba*)
BROME (*Bromus inermis*)
BERMUDAGRASS (*Cynodon dactylon*)
ORCHARDGRASS (*Dactylis glomerata*)
RYEGRASS (*Elymus & Lolium spp.*)
FESCUE (*Festuca elatior*)
TIMOTHY (*Phleum pratense*)
BLUEGRASS/JUNEGRASS (*Poa spp.*)

INDEX WEEDS: (Pollinating Season—Summer through Early Fall)
WATERHEMP (*Acnida tamariscina*)
PIGWEED (*Amaranthus retroflexus*)
SALTBUSH/SCALE (*Atriplex spp.*)
SUGARBEET (*Beta vulgaris*)
LAMB'S QUARTERS (*Chenopodium album*)
MEXICAN FIREBUSH (*Kochia scoparia*)
RUSSIAN THISTLE (*Salsola kali*)
RAGWEED, FALSE, GIANT, SHORT &
    WESTERN (*Ambrosia spp.*)
SAGEBRUSH (*Artemisia spp.*)
MARSH ELDER/POVERTY WEED (*Iva spp.*)
COCKLEBUR (*Xanthium strumarium*)
PLANTAIN (*Plantago lanceolata*)
DOCK/SORREL (*Rumex spp.*)

Region XII

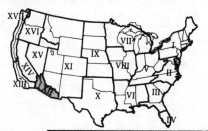

The Arid Southwest

Arizona   Southern California (S.E. Desert)

VEGETATION:

Trees — Creosote bush shrub and palo verde-cactus shrub; predominant trees cultivated.

Grasses — Several genera, naturalized and/or cultivated for hay and lawns wherever possible, although inconspicuous, are significant in hayfever.

Weeds — Although relatively few species of weeds are important, their widespread abundance and heavy pollination over a long season make them important hayfever plants. Many of these are shrubby relatives of weeds common to regions with more precipitation.

INDEX TREES: (Pollinating Season — Winter through Spring)
CYPRESS (*Cupressus arizonica*)
CEDAR/JUNIPER (*Juniperus californica*)
MESQUITE (*Prosopis juliflora*)
ASH (*Fraxinus velutina*)
OLIVE (*Olea europaea*)
COTTONWOOD/POPLAR (*Populus fremontii*)
ELM (*Ulmus parvifolia*)

INDEX GRASSES: (Pollinating Season — Spring through Early Summer)
BROME (*Bromus spp.*)
BERMUDAGRASS (*Cynodon dactylon*)
SALTGRASS (*Distichlis sp.*)
RYEGRASS (*Elymus & Lolium spp.*)
CANARYGRASS (*Phalaris minor*)
BLUEGRASS/JUNEGRASS (*Poa spp.*)

INDEX WEEDS: (Pollinating Season — Summer through Early Fall)
CARELESS WEED (*Amaranthus palmeri*)
IODINE BUSH (*Allenrolfea occidentalis*)
SALTBUSH/SCALE (*Atriplex spp.*)
LAMB'S QUARTERS (*Chenopodium album*)
RUSSIAN THISTLE (*Salsola kali*)
ALKALI-BLITE (*Suaeda sp.*)
RAGWEED, FALSE, SLENDER & WESTERN
   (*Ambrosia spp.*)
SAGEBRUSH (*Artemisia spp.*)
SILVER RAGWEED (*Dicoria canescens*)
BURRO BRUSH (*Hymenoclea salsola*)

Region XIII

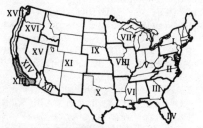

Southern Coastal California

STATES:
California, Southern Coastal

VEGETATION:

Trees—Chaparral and coastal sagebrush shrub to California steppe; many species of ornamental trees cultivated.

Grasses—Several genera, naturalized and/or cultivated for hay and lawns, although inconspicuous, are very abundant and significant in hayfever.

Weeds—Although relatively few species of weeds are important, their widespread abundance and heavy pollination over a long season make them important hayfever plants.

INDEX TREES: (Pollinating Season—Late Winter through Spring)
  BOX ELDER (*Acer negundo*)
  CYPRESS (*Cupressus arizonica*)
  OAK (*Quercus agrifolia*)
  WALNUT (*Juglans spp.*)
  ACACIA (*Acacia spp.*)
  MULBERRY (*Morus spp.*)
  EUCALYPTUS (*Eucalyptus sp.*)
  ASH (*Fraxinus velutina*)
  OLIVE (*Olea europaea*)
  SYCAMORE (*Platanus racemosa*)
  COTTONWOOD/POPLAR (*Populus trichocarpa*)
  ELM (*Ulmus spp.*)

INDEX GRASSES: (Pollinating Season—Spring through Early Summer)
  OATS (*Avena spp.*)
  BROME (*Bromus spp.*)
  BERMUDAGRASS (*Cynodon dactylon*)
  ORCHARDGRASS (*Dactylis glomerata*)
  SALTGRASS (*Distichlis sp.*)
  RYEGRASS (*Elymus & Lolium spp.*)
  FESCUE (*Festuca elatior*)
  BLUEGRASS/JUNEGRASS (*Poa spp.*)
  JOHNSONGRASS (*Sorghum halepense*)

Region XIV

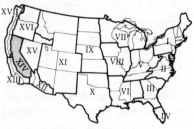

The Central California Valley

STATES:
   California (Sacramento and San Joaquin Valleys)

VEGETATION:
   Trees — California steppe bordered by California oakwoods; many species of ornamental, nut, and fruit trees cultivated.

   Grasses — Several genera, naturalized and/or cultivated for hay and lawns, although inconspicuous, are very abundant and significant in hayfever.

   Weeds — Although relatively few species of weeds are important, their widespread abundance and heavy pollination over a long season make them important hayfever plants.

INDEX GRASSES: (Pollinating Season—Spring through Early Summer)
REDTOP (*Agrostis alba*)
OATS (*Avena spp.*)
BROME (*Bromus spp.*)
BERMUDAGRASS (*Cynodon dactylon*)
ORCHARDGRASS (*Dactylis glomerata*)
SALTGRASS (*Distichlis sp.*)
RYEGRASS (*Elymus & Lolium spp.*)
FESCUE (*Festuca elatior*)
CANARYGRASS (*Phalaris minor*)
TIMOTHY (*Phleum pratense*)
BLUEGRASS/JUNEGRASS (*Poa spp.*)
JOHNSONGRASS (*Sorghum halepense*)

INDEX WEEDS: (Pollinating Season—Summer through Early Fall)
PIGWEED (*Amaranthus retroflexus*)
SALTBUSH/SCALE (*Atriplex spp.*)
SUGARBEET (*Beta vulgaris*)
LAMB'S QUARTERS (*Chenopodium album*)
RUSSIAN THISTLE (*Salsola kali*)
RAGWEED, FALSE, SLENDER & WESTERN
    (*Ambrosia spp.*)
SAGEBRUSH (*Artemisia spp.*)
COCKLEBUR (*Xanthium strumarium*)
PLANTAIN (*Plantago laceolata*)
DOCK/SORREL (*Rumex spp.*)

Region XV

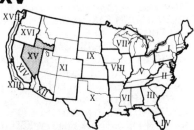

The Intermountain West

STATES:
Idaho (Southern)   Nevada

VEGETATION:
Trees—Sagebrush steppe, saltbush-greasewood and Great Basin sagebrush shrub; predominant trees cultivated.

Grasses—Several genera, naturalized and/or cultivated for hay and lawns wherever possible, although inconspicuous, are significant in hay-fever.

Weeds—Although relatively few species of weeds are important, their widespread abundance and heavy pollination over a long season make them important hayfever plants. Many of these are shrubby relatives of weeds common to regions with more precipitation.

INDEX TREES: (Pollinating Season—Late Winter through Spring)

BOX ELDER (*Acer negundo*)
ALDER (*Alnus incana*)
BIRCH (*Betula fontinalis*)
CEDAR/JUNIPER (*Juniperus utahensis*)
ASH (*Fraxinus americana*)
SYCAMORE (*Platanus occidentalis*)
COTTONWOOD/POPLAR (*Populus trichocarpa*)
ELM (*Ulmus spp.*)

INDEX GRASSES: (Pollinating Season—Spring through Early Summer)

QUACKGRASS/WHEATGRASS (*Agropyron spp.*)
REDTOP (*Agrostis alba*)
BROME (*Bromus inermis*)
BERMUDAGRASS (*Cynodon dactylon*)
ORCHARDGRASS (*Dactylis glomerata*)
SALTGRASS (*Distichlis sp.*)
RYEGRASS (*Elymus & Lolium spp.*)
FESCUE (*Festuca elatior*)
TIMOTHY (*Phleum pratense*)
BLUEGRASS/JUNEGRASS (*Poa spp.*)

INDEX WEEDS: (Pollinating Season—Summer through Early Fall)

PIGWEED (*Amaranthus retroflexus*)
IODINE BUSH (*Allenrolfea occidentalis*)
SALTBUSH/SCALE (*Atriplex spp.*)
LAMB'S QUARTERS (*Chenopodium album*)
MEXICAN FIREBUSH (*Kochia scoparia*)
RUSSIAN THISTLE (*Salsola kali*)
RAGWEED, FALSE, SLENDER &
    WESTERN (*Ambrosia spp.*)
SAGEBRUSH (*Artemisia spp.*)
MARSH ELDER/POVERTY WEED (*Iva spp.*)
COCKLEBUR (*Xanthium strumarium*)
PLANTAIN (*Plantago lanceolata*)
DOCK/SORREL (*Rumex spp.*)

Region XVI

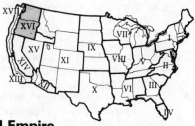

The Inland Empire

STATES:
Oregon (Central and Eastern)
Washington (Central and Eastern)

VEGETATION:

Trees—Bluegrass-fescue-wheatgrass grasslands and sagebrush steppe bordered by coniferous forests; predominant trees cultivated.

Grasses—This region is predominantly grassland, but the more important hayfever grasses are cultivated for seed, hay, or lawns, or are naturalized pests.

Weeds—Although relatively few species of weeds are important, their widespread abundance and heavy pollination over a long season make them important hayfever plants.

INDEX TREES: (Pollinating Season—Late Winter through Spring)
BOX ELDER (*Acer negundo*)
ALDER (*Alnus incana*)
BIRCH (*Betula fontinalis*)
OAK (*Quercus garryana*)
WALNUT (*Juglans nigra*)
PINE (*Pinus spp.*)
COTTONWOOD/POPLAR (*Populus trichocarpa*)
WILLOW (*Salix lasiandra*)

INDEX GRASSES: (Pollinating Season—Spring through Early Summer)
QUACKGRASS/WHEATGRASS (*Agropyron spp.*)
REDTOP (*Agrostis alba*)
VERNALGRASS (*Anthoxanthum sp.*)
BROME (*Bromus inermis*)
ORCHARDGRASS (*Dactylis glomerata*)
RYEGRASS (*Elymus & Lolium spp.*)
VELVETGRASS (*Holcus lanatus*)
TIMOTHY (*Phleum pratense*)
BLUEGRASS/JUNEGRASS (*Poa spp.*)

INDEX WEEDS: (Pollinating Season—Summer through Early Fall)
  PIGWEED (*Amaranthus retroflexus*)
  SALTBUSH/SCALE (*Atriplex spp.*)
  LAMB'S QUARTERS (*Chenopodium album*)
  MEXICAN FIREBUSH (*Kochia scoparia*)
  RUSSIAN THISTLE (*Salsola kali*)
  RAGWEED, FALSE, GIANT, SHORT & WESTERN (*Ambrosia spp.*)
  SAGEBRUSH (*Artemisia spp.*)
  MARSH ELDER/POVERTY WEED (*Iva spp.*)
  PLANTAIN (*Plantago lanceolata*)
  DOCK/SORREL (*Rumex spp.*)

Region XVII

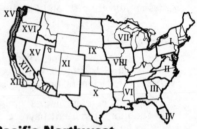

Cascade Pacific Northwest

STATES:
  California (Northwestern)   Oregon (Western)
  Washington (Western)

VEGETATION:
Trees—Mixed coniferous forests; hardwoods primarily cultivated.

Grasses—Several genera, naturalized and/or cultivated for hay and lawns, although inconspicuous, are very abundant and significant in hayfever. Grass seed is produced extensively in parts of this region.

Weeds—Although relatively few species of weeds are important, their widespread abundance and heavy pollination over a long season make them important hayfever plants.

INDEX TREES: (Pollinating Season—Late Winter through Spring)
  BOX ELDER (*Acer negundo*)
  ALDER (*Alnus rhombifolia*)
  BIRCH (*Betula fontinalis*)
  HAZELNUT (*Corylus cornuta*)
  OAK (*Quercus garryana*)
  WALNUT (*Juglans regia*)
  ASH (*Fraxinus oregona*)
  COTTONWOOD/POPLAR (*Populus trichocarpa*)
  WILLOW (*Salix lasiandra*)
  ELM (*Ulmus pumila*)

INDEX GRASSES: (Pollinating Season—Spring through Early Summer)
  BENTGRASS (*Agrostis maritima*)
  VERNALGRASS (*Anthoxanthum sp.*)
  OATS (*Avena spp.*)
  BROME (*Bromus inermis*)
  BERMUDAGRASS (*Cynodon dactylon*)
  ORCHARDGRASS (*Dactylis glomerata*)
  SALTGRASS (*Distichlis sp.*)
  RYEGRASS (*Elymus & Lolium spp.*)
  FESCUE (*Festuca elatior*)
  VELVETGRASS (*Holcus lanatus*)
  CANARYGRASS (*Phalaris arundinacea*)
  TIMOTHY (*Phleum pratense*)
  BLUEGRASS/JUNEGRASS (*Poa spp.*)

INDEX WEEDS: (Pollinating Season—Summer through Early Fall)
  PIGWEED (*Amaranthus retroflexus*)
  SALTBUSH/SCALE (*Atriplex spp.*)
  LAMB'S QUARTERS (*Chenopodium album*)
  RUSSIAN THISTLE (*Salsola kali*)
  RAGWEED, FALSE, GIANT, SHORT &
    WESTERN (*Ambrosia spp.*)
  SAGEBRUSH (*Artemisia spp.*)
  COCKELBUR (*Xanthium strumarium*)
  PLANTAIN (*Plantago lanceolata*)
  DOCK/SORREL (*Rumex spp.*)

Region C-I

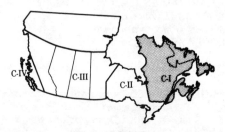

Atlantic Provinces & Quebec

PROVINCES:

Prince Edward Island   Nova Scotia
New Brunswick   Newfoundland
Quebec

VEGETATION:

Trees—From south to north, mixed wood forests and boreal forests open into woodlands and tundras through Quebec and Newfoundland, Acadian forests in the other Provinces.

Grasses—Several genera, naturalized and/or cultivated for hay and lawns, are very abundant and more significant than the native grasses in hayfever.

Weeds—Although relatively few species of weeds are important, their abundance in agricultural and urban areas makes them important hayfever plants.

INDEX TREES: (Pollinating Season—Late Winter through Spring)
BOX ELDER (Manitoba Maple) (*Acer negundo*)
HARD MAPLE (Sugar) (*Acer saccharum*)
TAG ALDER (Speckled) (*Alnus incana*)
PAPER BIRCH (White) (*Betula papyrifera*)
BEECH (*Fagus grandifolia*)
WHITE ASH (*Fraxinus americana*)
GREEN ASH (*Fraxinus pennsylvanica*)
BUTTERNUT (*Juglans cinerea*)
SYCAMORE (*Platanus occidentalis*)
BALSAM POPLAR (*Populus balsamifera*)
TREMBLING ASPEN (*Populus tremuloides*)
BUR OAK (*Quercus macrocarpa*)
BLACK WILLOW (*Salix nigra*)
AMERICAN ELM (White) (*Ulmus americana*)

INDEX GRASSES: (Pollinating Season—Spring through Early Summer)
QUACKGRASS (Couch) (*Agropyron repens*)
REDTOP (*Agrostis alba*)
BROME (*Bromus sp.*)
ORCHARDGRASS (*Dactylis glomerata*)
RYEGRASS (*Elymus/Lolium spp.*)
TIMOTHY (*Phleum pratense*)
BLUEGRASS (*Poa spp.*)

INDEX WEEDS: (Pollinating Season—Summer through Early Fall)
REDROOT PIGWEED (*Amaranthus retroflexus*)
RAGWEED (*Ambrosia spp.*)
LAMB'S QUARTERS (*Chenopodium album*)
PLANTAIN (*Plantago lanceolata*)
DOCK/SORREL (*Rumex spp.*)
RUSSIAN THISTLE (*Salsola kali*)

Region C-II

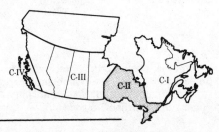

PROVINCE:
Ontario

VEGETATION:
Trees—From south to north, mixed wood forests and boreal forests open into woodlands and tundras.

Grasses—Several genera, naturalized and/or cultivated for hay and lawns, are very abundant and more significant than the native grasses in hayfever.

Weeds—Although relatively few species of weeds are important, their abundance in agricultural and urban areas makes them important hayfever plants.

INDEX TREES: (Pollinating Season—Late Winter through Spring)
BOX ELDER (Manitoba Maple) (*Acer negundo*)
HARD MAPLE (Sugar) (*Acer saccharum*)
TAG ALDER (Speckled) (*Alnus incana*)
PAPER BIRCH (White) (*Betula papyrifera*)
BEECH (*Fagus grandifolia*)
WHITE ASH (*Fraxinus americana*)
GREEN ASH (*Fraxinus pennsylvanica*)
BUTTERNUT (*Juglans cinerea*)
SYCAMORE (*Platanus occidentalis*)
BALSAM POPLAR (*Populus balsamifera*)
ASPEN (*Populus tremuloides*)
BUR OAK (*Quercus macrocarpa*)
BLACK WILLOW (*Salix nigra*)
AMERICAN ELM (White) (*Ulmus americana*)
CHINESE ELM (Siberian) (*Ulmus pumila*)

INDEX GRASSES: (Pollinating Season—Spring through Early Summer)
QUACKGRASS (Couch) (*Agropyron repens*)
REDTOP (*Agrostis alba*)
BROME (*Bromus sp.*)
ORCHARDGRASS (*Dactylis glomerata*)
RYEGRASS (*Elymus/Lolium spp.*)
TIMOTHY (*Phleum pratense*)
BLUEGRASS (*Poa spp.*)

INDEX WEEDS: (Pollinating Season—Summer through Early Fall)
REDROOT PIGWEED (*Amaranthus retroflexus*)
RAGWEED (*Ambrosia spp.*)
LAMB'S QUARTERS (*Chenopodium album*)
ENGLISH PLANTAIN (*Plantago lanceolata*)
DOCK/SORREL (*Rumex spp.*)
RUSSIAN THISTLE (*Salsola kali*)

Region C-III

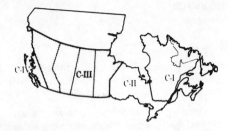

Prairie Provinces and
Eastern British Columbia

PROVINCES:

Alberta
Manitoba

Eastern British Columbia
Saskatchewan

VEGETATION:

Trees — The southern third of the region is grass-land and parkland, where the predominant trees are found only along watercourses or are culti-vated. Cordilleran forests are in the west, mixed wood forests in the north, and boreal forests in the northern most parts.

Grasses — The more populous part of this region is predominately grassland, but the more impor-tant hayfever grasses are cultivated for hay or lawns, or are naturalized pests.

Weeds — Although relatively few species of weeds are important in Canada, there are several more species in this region; their abundance in agricultural and urban areas making them impor-tant hayfever plants.

INDEX TREES: (Pollinating Season — Late Winter through Spring)

BOX ELDER (Manitoba maple) (*Acer negundo*)
TAG ALDER (Speckled-Mountain) (*Alnus incana*)
PAPER BIRCH (White) (*Betula papyrifera*)
GREEN ASH (*Fraxinus pennsylvanica*)
BALSAM POPLAR (*Populus balsamifera*)
TREMBLING ASPEN (*Populus tremuloides*)
BUR OAK (*Quercus macrocarpa*)
WILLOW (Yellow) (*Salix sp.*)
CHINESE ELM (Siberian) (*Ulmus pumila*)

INDEX GRASSES: (Pollinating Season — Spring through Early Summer)

QUACKGRASS (Couch) WHEATGRASS
(*Agropyron spp.*)
REDTOP (*Agrostis alba*)
COMMON WILD OATS (*Avena fatua*)
BROME (*Bromus sp.*)

ORCHARD GRASS (*Dactylis glomerata*)
RYEGRASS (*Elymus/Lolium spp.*)
TIMOTHY (*Phleum pratense*)
BLUEGRASS (*Poa spp.*)

INDEX WEEDS: (Pollinating Season — Summer through Early Fall)
REDROOT PIGWEED (*Amaranthus retroflexus*)
RAGWEED (*Ambrosia spp.*)
LAMB'S QUARTERS (*Chenopodium album*)
SAGEBRUSH (*Artemisia spp.*)
MARSHELDER/POVERTY WEED (*Iva spp.*)
ENGLISH PLANTAIN (*Plantago lanceolata*)
DOCK/SORREL (*Rumex spp.*)
RUSSIAN THISTLE (*Salsola kali*)

Region C-IV

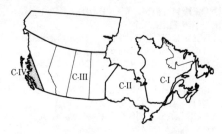

Western British Columbia & Vancouver Island

PROVINCES:
Western British Columbia   Vancouver Island

VEGETATION:
Trees — Except for the steppe, where the predominant trees are found only along watercourses or are cultivated, this region is cordilleran forest.

Grasses — Several genera, naturalized and/or cultivated for hay and lawns, are very abundant and more significant than the native grasses in hayfever.

Weeds — Although relatively few species of weeds are important, their abundance in agricultural and urban areas makes them important hayfever plants.

INDEX TREES: (Pollinating Season — Late Winter through Spring)
BOX ELDER (Manitoba Maple) (*Acer negundo*)
RED ALDER (*Alnus rubra*)
SITKA ALDER (*Alnus sinuata*)
PAPER BIRCH (White) (*Betula papyrifera*)
SYCAMORE (*Platanus occidentalis*)
BLACK COTTONWOOD (*Populus trichocarpa*)

TREMBLING ASPEN (*Populus tremuloides*)
DOUGLAS FIR (*Pseudotsuga menziesii*)
GARRY'S OAK (*Quercus garryana*)
YELLOW WILLOW (Pacific) (*Salix lasiandra*)
CHINESE ELM (Siberian) (*Ulmus pumila*)

INDEX GRASSES: (Pollinating Season – Spring through Early Summer)
QUACKGRASS (Couch) (*Agropyron repens*)
REDTOP (*Agrostis alba*)
TALL OAT GRASS (*Arrhenatherum elatius*)
COMMON WILD OATS (*Avena fatua*)
BROME (*Bromus sp.*)
ORCHARDGRASS (*Dactylis glomerata*)
RYEGRASS (*Elymus/Lolium spp.*)
TIMOTHY (*Phleum pratense*)
BLUEGRASS (*Poa spp.*)

INDEX WEEDS: (Pollinating Season – Summer through Early Fall)
REDROOT PIGWEED (*Amaranthus retroflexus*)
RAGWEED (*Ambrosia spp.*)
LAMB'S QUARTERS (*Chenopodium album*)
MARSHELDER/POVERTY WEED (*Iva spp.*)
ENGLISH PLANTAIN (*Plantago lanceolata*)
DOCK/SORREL (*Rumex spp.*)
RUSSIAN THISTLE (*Salsola kali*)

Region: Alaska

Alaska
STATE:
Alaska
VEGETATION:
Typical hayfever species of the three plant forms, viz. trees, grasses, and weeds, are found in the southern coastal region which forms an arc from the southeasternmost point of the state northward, westward, then southward to the Alaska Peninsula. As a whole, the state has three principal vegetation types:
1. Dense sitka spruce and western hemlock forests. These trees are generally considered of very minor significance in allergy, if significant at all. However, alder, aspen, birch, and willow may be found in clearings and near watercourses, and may be associated with grasses and some weeds in the early stages of plant succession.
2. Less dense forests of birches and white spruce. The birches may be the most significant hayfever trees because they form such extensive forests.
3. Tundra and tundra-like, characterized by low vegetation, in the Aleutian Islands, the Bering Sea Coast and the Arctic Slope. Very

cold winters and very cool moist summers are detrimental to tree growth. Grasses are predominant, but (as in tropical regions) the humidity and precipitation are so great that whatever airborne pollen is shed is not likely to remain airborne very long.

Index grasses and weeds are most common in the temperate agricultural and urban regions. The whole hayfever season is short, from three to six months according to lattitude, elevation, and proximity to the seacoasts.

INDEX TREES: (Pollinating Season — Spring)
ALDER (*Alnus incana*)
ASPEN (*Populus tremuloides*)
BIRCH (*Betula papyrifera*)
CEDAR (*Thuja plicata*)
HEMLOCK (*Tsuga hetrophylla*)
PINE (*Pinus contorta*)
POPLAR (*Populus balsamifera*)
SPRUCE (*Picea sitchensis*)
WILLOW (*Salix spp.*)

INDEX GRASSES: (Pollinating Season — Late Spring-Summer)
BLUEGRASS/JUNEGRASS (*Poa spp.*)
BROME (*Bromus inermis*)
CANARYGRASS (*Phalaris arundinacea*)
FESCUE (*Festuca rubra*)
ORCHARDGRASS (*Dactylis glomerata*)
QUACKGRASS/WHEATGRASS (*Agropyron spp.*)
REDTOP (*Agrostis alba*)
RYEGRASS (*Lolium perenne*)
TIMOTHY (*Phleum pratense*)

INDEX WEEDS: (Pollinating Season — Summer)
BULRUSH (*Scirpus spp.*)
DOCK/SORREL (*Rumex spp.*)
LAMB'S QUARTERS (*Chenopodium album*)
NETTLE (*Urtica dioica*)
PLANTAIN (*Plantago lanceolata*)
SAGEBRUSH/WORMWOOD (*Artemisa spp.*)
SEDGE (*Carex spp.*)
SPEARSCALE (*Atriplex patula*)

Region: Hawaii (all islands)

Hawaii

STATE:
Hawaii

VEGETATION:
Although Hawaii is small in total land surface, it has a wide range of habitats which vary from dense tropical forests to virtually barren mountaintops, from wet windward parts of islands to dry scrub land in the rain shadows. Consequent-

ly, the vegetation is extremely varied and complex, changing abruptly within short distances.

The seasonality of hayfever is less defined because the major agricultural and urban centers enjoy virtually a continuous growing season. Grasses and annual weeds may be flowering all year with one or few peak periods.

The long growing season and diversity of habitats create optimum situations for the establishment of newly introduced species; both deliberate and accidental. (Man has introduced, for example, some 500 species of grasses alone—one family!) Entomophilous (insect vector) flowers abound; although they produce relatively little pollen per individual flower, their sheer abundance and widespread use may make them more important than would be expected according to Thommen's postulates. The enormous task of identifying, collecting, and purifying these pollens for clinical testing and assessing is still in developmental stages.

Pollinating Season: Less defined than continental regions.

INDEX TREES:
ACACIA (*Acacia spp.*)
AUSTRALIAN PINE (BEEFWOOD) (*Casuarina equisetifolia*)
CEDAR/JUNIPER (*Juniperus spp.*)
MONTERY CYPRESS (*Cupressus macrocarpa*)
DATE PALM (*Phoenix dactylifera*)
EUCALYPTUS (GUM) (*Eucalyptus globulus*)
MESQUITE (*Prosopis juliflora*)
PAPER MULBERRY (*Broussonetia papyrifera*)
OLIVE (*Olea europaea*)
PRIVET (*Ligustrum spp.*)

INDEX GRASSES:
BERMUDAGRASS (*Cynodon dactylon*)
CORN (*Zea mays*)
FINGERGRASS (*Chloris spp.*)
JOHNSONGRASS (*Sorghum halepense*)
LOVEGRASS (*Eragrostis spp.*)
BLUEGRASS/JUNEGRASS (*Poa spp.*)
REDTOP (*Agrostis alba*)
SORGHUM (*Sorghum vulgare*)

INDEX WEEDS:
COCKLEBUR (*Xanthium strumarium*)
PLANTAIN (*Plantago lanceolata*)
KOCHIA (*Kochia scoparia*)
PIGWEED (*Amaranthus spp.*)
RAGWEED, SLENDER (*Ambrosia sp.*)
SAGEBRUSH (*Artemisia spp.*)
SCALE (SALTBUSH) (*Atriplex spp.*)

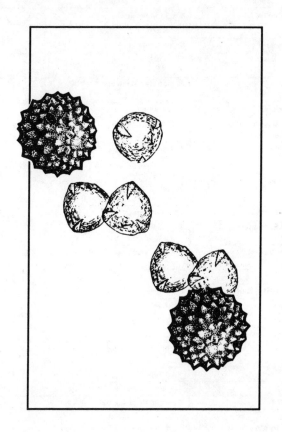

A Classification of Significant Hayfever
TREES, GRASSES, WEEDS AND CULTIVATED PLANTS

Name: Common	Name: Technical	Plant Form	Family
ACACIA, Bailey's	Acacia baileyana	T	Leguminosae
ACACIA	A. decurrens	T	"
ACACIA, Longleaf	A. longifolia	T	"
ALDER, Red (Oregon)	Alnus rubra	T	Betulaceae
ALDER, Sitka	A. sinuata (A. sitchensis)	T	"
ALDER, Slender	A. tenuifolia	T	"
ALDER, Tag (Speckled)	A. incana (A. rugosa)	T	"
ALDER, White	A. rhombifolia	T	"
ALFALFA	Medicago sativa	W	Leguminosae
ALLSCALE	Atriplex polycarpa	W	Chenopodiaceae
ARBOR-VITAE, Chinese	Thuja orientalis	T	Cupressaceae
ARBOR-VITAE, Western (White Cedar)	T. occidentalis	T	"
ASH (Arizona Velvet)	Fraxinus velutina	T	Oleaceae
ASH, Black	F. nigra	T	"
ASH, Green (ASH, Red)	F. pennsylvanica	T	"
ASH, Mexican	F. uhdei	T	"
ASH, Oregon	F. oregona	T	"
ASH, White	F. americana	T	"
ASPEN	Populus tremuloides	T	Salicaceae
ASTER	Aster spp.	W	Compositae
BAHIAGRASS	Paspalum notatum	G	Gramineae
BALSAMROOT	Balsamorrhiza sagittata	W	Compositae
BARLEY, Cultivated	Hordeum vulgare	G	Gramineae
BARLEY, Wall	H. murinum	G	"
BARNYARDGRASS	Echinochloa crusgalli	G	Gramineae
BASSIA	Bassia hyssopifolia	W	Chenopodiaceae
BEACHBUR	Franseria bipinnatifida	W	Compositae
BEACHBUR, San Francisco	F. chamissonis	W	"
BEECH, American	Fagus grandifolia	T	Fagaceae
BEEFWOOD (AUSTRAL. PINE)	Casuarina equisetifolia	T	Casuarinaceae
BEET	Beta vulgaris	W	Chenopodiaceae

Key To Alphabetical Code

A Major Importance   T Trees
B Medium Importance   G Grasses
C Minor Importance   W Weeds

Distribution	Pollination Period	Importance		
		Allergenic	Plant	Pollen
Cultivated ornamental (Subtropical)	Mar.-May	C	C	C
Cultivated ornamental (Subtropical)	Mar.-May	C	C	C
Cultivated ornamental (Subtropical)	Mar.-May	C	C	C
Pacific Coast from S.W. YT. to S. CA., rarely more than 50 mi. from salt or over 2500' elev.	Mar.-Apr.	B	B	A
AK. S. to Olympic Mts., Cascade Mts., N. CA., E. WA., N.E. OR., Rocky Mts.	May-July	B	B	A
N.E. MN., ND. to BC., S. to NM.	Mar.-May	B	B	A
NF. to NWT. and BC., S. to MD., N. to IN. and MN., MT., ID., WA.	Mar.-May	B	B	A
N. ID. to E. slope Cascades, to S. OR., W. slope of Sierra Nevada, S. to Coast Range in CA.	Jan.-Apr.	B	B	A
Cultivated crop	May-Oct.	C	C	C
Colorado and Mohave Desert, Alkali Flats of C. CA., S. NV., UT., and AZ.	July-Oct.	A	A	A
Cultivated ornamental	Apr.-May	C	C	B
PQ. and NS. to Hudson Bay, S. to NJ., OH., N. IN. and IL., WI., MN., Mts. NC. and TN.	Apr.-May	C	B	B
CA., AZ., S. NM., E. TX. Cultivated in these areas	Mar.-Apr.	B	B	B
NF. and PQ. to MAN., S. to DE., KY., IA.	Spring	B	B	B
PQ. to MAN., S. to FL. and TX.	Spring	B	B	B
Cultivated ornamental	Winter	C	C	C
C. CA. N. to BC.	Mar.-May	B	B	B
NS. to MN., S. to FL. and TX.	Spring	B	B	B
LAB. to AK., S. to NJ., VA., TN., MO., Rocky Mts., Sierra Nevada, Cascades	Apr.-June	B	B	B
Cultivated ornamentals and native weeds	July-Oct.	C	C	C
S.E. US.	May-Nov.	B	A	B
S. BC. to S. CA., E. to MT., SD., CO.	Apr.-July	C	C	C
Cultivated	Jan. (May-June) Dec.	C	C	C
S. BC., W. WA.	June-July	C	C	C
Widespread weed	June-Oct.	C	B	C
BC. to CA., E. to MT., ID., NV., spreading elsewhere	July-Oct.	B	B	B
Coastal beaches and dunes BC. to S. CA.	Mar.-Sept.	B	B	B
Coastal beaches and dunes BC. to S. CA.	July-Sept.	B	B	B
NS. to MN., S. to FL. and TX.	Spring	C	B	C
Cultivated ornamental (Subtropical)	Jan.-Mar.	B	B	B
Cultivated crop (Sugar and Red) established locally in S. US.	July-Oct.	B	B	B

Name: Common	Name: Technical	Plant Form	Family
BENTGRASS	Agrostis maritima	G	Gramineae
BERMUDAGRASS	Cynodon dactylon	G	Gramineae
BIRCH, Cherry (Black)	Betula lenta	T	Betulaceae
BIRCH, European White	B. pendula alba	T	,,
BIRCH, Paperbark	B. papyrifera	T	,,
BIRCH, River (Red)	B. nigra	T	,,
BIRCH, Spring	B. fontinalis	T	,,
BIRCH, Yellow	B. lutea	T	,,
BLUEGRASS, Annual	Poa annua	G	Gramineae
BLUEGRASS, Canada	P. compressa	G	,,
BLUEGRASS, Kentucky	P. pratensis	G	,,
BLUEGRASS, Pine	P. scabrella	G	,,
BLUEGRASS, Sandberg	P. sandbergii	G	,,
BLUEGRASS, Shady (Rough)	P. trivialis	G	,,
BOTTLEBRUSH	Calistemon spp.	T	Myrtaceae
BOX ELDER (Ash-leaved Maple, Manitoba Maple)	Acer negundo	T	Aceraceae
BRACTSCALE	Atriplex bracteosa	W	Chenopodiaceae
BREWERS SCALE	A. breweri	W	,,
BRITTLE BUSH (Incienso)	Encelia farinosa	W	Compositae
SCOTCH BROOM	Cystisus scoparius	W	Leguminosae
BROOMWEED	Gutierrezia dracunculoides	W	Compositae
BROME, California	Bromus carinatus	G	Gramineae
BROME, Mountain	B. marginatus	G	,,
BROME, Smooth	B. inermis	G	,,
BROME, Soft (Soft Cheat)	B. hordeaceus (B. mollis)	G	,,
BULRUSH	Scirpus microcarpus	W	Cyperaceae
BUNCHGRASS, Northwest	Agropyron spicatum	G	Gramineae
BURROBRUSH	Hymenoclea monogyra	W	Compositae
BURROBRUSH	H. salsola	W	,,
BUTTERNUT (White Walnut)	Juglans cinerea	T	Juglandaceae
CANE, Sugar	Saccharum officinarum	G	Gramineae
CANAIGRE (Wild Rhubarb)	Rumex hymenosepalus	W	Polygonaceae
CANARYGRASS, Common	Phalaris canariensis	G	Gramineae
CANARYGRASS, Little	P. minor	G	,,
CANARYGRASS, Reed	P. arundinacea	G	,,

Distribution	Pollination Period	Importance		
		Aller-genic	Plant	Pollen
Widespread in Canada and US.	June-Sept.	A	A	A
Cultivated lawn grass, S. US., locally farther north	Jan. (June-Sept.) Dec.	A	A	A
IA., S. ME. and S.W. PQ. to DE. and KY., along Appalachians to GA.	Mar.-May	B	B	B
Cultivated ornamental	Mar.-May	B	B	B
LAB. to Ak., S. to NJ. WV., N. IN., N.E. IA., W. to MT., WA.	Mar.-May	B	B	B
NH. to FL., W. to S. OH., S. MI., S.E. MN., E. KS., and TX.	Feb.-June	B	B	B
AK. to CA., E. to SASK., ND., SD., Rocky Mt. States	Feb.-June	B	B	B
NFLD. to MAN., S. to DE., PA., N. OH., N. IN., N.E. IA., along Appalachians to GA.	Spring	B	B	B
Widespread weed	Jan. (Mar.-Aug.) Dec.	A	A	A
NFLD. to AK., S. throughout most of US.	June-Aug.	A	A	A
Cultivated lawn grass, temperate Canada, all but S.E. US.	May-Oct.	A	A	A
YT. to BC., S. to CA., E. to ALTA., MI, MN., WY., CO.	Apr.-July	A	A	A
YT. to BC. S. to CA., NV., E. to SASK., ND., SD., NB., CO., NM.	Apr.-Aug.	A	A	A
E. Canada and N.E. US., AK. to CA.	May-July	A	A	A
Cultivated ornamental (Subtropical)	All Seasons	C	C	C
S. Canada, VT. to FL., W. nearly to Pacific Coast	Mar.-May	B	B	B
C. and S. CA., E. to NM., TX.	July-Nov.	A	A	A
C. and S. CA.	July-Oct.	A	A	A
C. and S. CA., to S.W. UT., AZ.	Mar.-May	C	C	C
Naturalized, CA., N. to WA., BC.	Apr.-June	C	C	C
C. TX. and OK.	July-Oct.	C	B	C
AK. to S. CA., E. to ALTA., ND., SD., WY., CO., NM., introduced locally farther E.	Apr.-Aug.	B	A	B
BC. to CA., E. to SD., NM.	Apr.-July	B	A	B
AK. to CA., introduced to LAB., VT., OH., NM., Rocky Mts. S. to CO.	June-Aug.	A	A	A
AK. to S. CA., E. to ID. and MT.	May-July	B	A	B
S. CA., N. to Ak., Rocky Mts., NM.	May-Aug.	C	C	C
AK. to CA., E. to ATLA., ND., SD., NM.	June-Aug.	B	B	B
S. CO. E. to TX.	Aug.-Nov.	A	A	A
S. CA., NV., S. UT., AZ.	Mar.-June	A	A	A
Cultivated ornamental and native tree, NB. to ONT., N. MI., ND., S. to VA., GA., AR., KS.	Apr.-May	B	B	B
Cultivated crop	Rarely allowed to flower	C	C	C
C. and S. CA., WY., W. TX.	Jan.-May	C	C	B
WA. to CA., Rocky Mt. States, E. to Atlantic Coast	June-Aug.	B	B	B
OR. to CA., Atlantic Coast	Apr.-July	B	B	B
S. AK. and Canada, all but S.E. US.	June-July	B	B	B

Name: Common	Name: Technical	Plant Form	Family
CARELESSWEED	Amaranthus palmeri	W	Amaranthaceae
CAROB	Ceratonia siliqua	T	Leguminosae
CASTOR BEAN	Ricinus communis	W	Euphorbiaceae
CATTAIL, Broad-leaf	Typha latifolia	W	Typhaceae
CATTAIL, Narrow-leaf	T. angustifolia	W	''
CEDAR, Atlantic	Cedrus atlantica	T	Pinaceae
CEDAR, Deodar	C. deodara	T	''
CEDAR, Giant (Canoe)	Thuja plicata	T	Cupressaceae
CEDAR, Incense	Libocedrus decurrens	T	Cupressaceae
CEDAR, Japanese	Cryptomeria japonica	T	Taxodiaceae
CEDAR, Salt	Tamarix gallica	T	Tamaricaceae
CHAMISE (Greasewood)	Adenostoma fasciculatum	W	Rosaceae
CHEAT (Chess)	Bromus secalinus	G	Gramineae
CHERRY	Prunus cerasus	T	Rosaceae
CHESTNUT, American	Castanea dentata	T	Fagaceae
CHESTNUT, Horse	Aesculus hippocastanum	T	Hippocastanaceae
CLOVER, Red	Trifolium pratense	W	Leguminosae
CLOVER, Sweet	Melilotus spp.	W	Leguminosae
CLOVER, White	Trifolium repens	W	Leguminosae
COCKLEBUR, Common	Xanthium strumarium	W	Compositae
COCKLEBUR, Spiny	X. spinosum	W	''
CORN	Zea mays	G	Gramineae
COTTONWOOD, Black	Populus trichocarpa	T	Salicaceae
COTTONWOOD, Eastern, (Carolina Poplar)	P. deltoides (includes P. sargentii)	T	Salicaceae
COTTONWOOD, Fremont	P. fremontii	T	''
CYPRESS, Arizona	Cupressus arizonica	T	Cuppressaceae
CYPRESS, Bald	Taxodium distichum	T	Taxodiaceae
CYPRESS, Italian	Cupressus sempervirens	T	Cupressaceae
CYPRESS, Monterey	Cupressus macrocarpa	T	Cupressaceae
DAISY, Ox-eye	Chrysanthemum leucantheum	W	Compositae
DALLISGRASS	Paspalun dilatatum	G	Gramineae
DANDELION	Taraxacum officinale	W	Compositae
DARNEL	Lolium temulentum	G	Gramineae
DOCK, Bitter	Rumex obtrusifolius	W	Polygonaceae
DOCK, Green	R. conglomeratus	W	''
DOCK, White	R. mexicanus	W	''
DOCK, Yellow (Curly Dock)	R. crispus	W	''
DOG FENNEL (Mayweed)	Anthemis cotula	W	Compositae
DROPSEED	Sporobolus airoides	G	Gramineae
DROPSEED, Sand	S. cryptandrus	G	''
ELDERBERRY	Sambucus glauca	T	Sambucaceae
ELM, American (White Elm)	Ulmus americana	T	Ulmaceae

Distribution	Pollination Period	Importance		
		Aller-genic	Plant	Pollen
S. CA., E. to C. US.	Aug.-Nov.	A	A	A
Cultivated ornamental	Late Winter Early Spring	C	C	C
Cultivated ornamental, established in S. US.	Jan.-Dec.	C	C	A
Widespread weed	June-Aug.	C	C	B
Widespread weed	June-Aug.	C	C	B
Cultivated ornamental	Winter	C	C	B
Cultivated ornamental	Winter	C	C	B
AK. to C. CA., W. MT.	Apr.-May	C	C	C
CA. to N. OR., W. to NV.	Apr.-May	C	C	C
Cultivated ornamental	Spring	C	C	C
Introduced, common in alkali western soils, along water courses	Mar.-Aug.	C	C	C
Common component of California Chaparral	May-June	C	C	C
Occasional throughout temperate N. America	June-July	C	B	C
Cultivated crop and ornamental	Mar.-May	C	C	C
Appalachia. Rare, nearly exterminated by blight	Spring	C	C	B
Cultivated ornamental	May-June	C	C	C
Cultivated hay crop	June-Aug.	C	C	C
Cultivated hay crop, widespread weed	May-Nov.	C	C	C
Cultivated lawn plant	Apr.-Sept.	C	C	C
Widespread weed	Aug.-Oct.	A	A	A
Widespread weed in warm and temperate regions	July-Oct.	B	B	A
Cultivated crop	Jan.-Dec.	B	B	B
S. CA. to AK., MT., ID., NV.	Feb.-Apr.	B	B	B
PQ. and New England to S. MAN., MN., to Rocky Mts., S. to FL. and TX.	Mar.-Apr.	B	B	B
C. and S. CA. to NV., AZ.	Mar.-Apr.	B	B	B
Native to AZ. and E. NM. Cultivated in CO. and S.W.	Mar.-Apr.	B	B	B
DE. to FL., W. to IL., MO., AR., and TX.	Spring	C	B	C
Cultivated ornamental	Feb.-Mar.	C	C	C
Monterey Peninsula	Spring	C	C	B
Widespread weed, cultivated as Shasta Daisy	June-Aug.	C	C	C
S. US. N. to NJ., TN., AR., OK., OR.	Spring-Fall	C	B	C
Widespread weed	Jan.-Dec.	C	A	C
From Europe, now naturalized in CA.	Apr.-June	B	C	A
Widespread weed	June-Dec.	B	B	A
Widespread weed	Apr.-Oct.	B	B	A
Widespread weed	June-Sept.	B	B	A
Widespread weed	May-Oct.	A	A	A
Widespread weed	June-Oct.	C	A	C
WA. to S. CA., SD., TX.	Apr.-Oct.	C	C	B
S. CA. to Atlantic Coast, LA.	May-Aug.	C	C	B
S. CA. to BC., ALTA., ID.	June-Sept.	C	B	C
NFLD. to MAN., S. to FL. and TX., also cultivated	Feb.-Apr.	B	B	B

Name: Common	Name: Technical	Plant Form	Family
ELM, Chinese	U. parvifolia	T	"
ELM, Fall-blooming (Cedar Elm)	U. crassifolia	T	"
ELM, Siberian (Chinese)	Ulmus pumila	T	"
ELM, Slippery (Red Elm)	U. fulva	T	"
FERN, Bracken	Pterdium aquilinum	W	Dennstaedtiaceae
FERN, Sword (Christmas Fern)	Polystichum munitum	W	Polypodiaceae
FERN, Royal	Osmunda regalis	W	Osmundaceae
FESCUE, Meadow	Festuca elatior	G	Gramineae
FESCUE, Red	F. rubra	G	"
FESCUE, Sheep	F. ovina	G	"
FIR, Douglas	Pseudotsuga menziesii	T	Pinaceae
FIR, Noble (Red)	Abies nobilis	T	Pinaceae
FIR, White	A. concolor	T	"
FIREBUSH, Mex. (Smr. Cypress)	Kochia scoparia	W	Chenopodiaceae
FIREWEED (Willow-herb)	Epilobium angustifolium	W	Onagraceae
GAMAGRASS	Tripsacum dactyloides	G	Gramineae
GOLDENROD	Solidago spp.	W	Compositae
GOOSEFOOT, Nettle-leaf	Chenopodium murale	W	Chenopodiaceae
GRAMAGRASS	Bouteloua spp.	G	Gramineae
GREASEWOOD	Sarcobatus vermiculatus	W	Chenopodiaceae
GUM, Blue	Eucalyptus globulus	T	Myrtaceae
GUM, Sweet	Liquidambar styraciflua	T	Altingiaceae
HACKBERRY	Celtis occidentalis	T	Ulmaceae
HAZLENUT, American	Corylus americana	T	Corylaceae
HAZLENUT, Beaked	Corylus cornuta	T	"
HEMLOCK, Canada (Eastern)	Tsuga canadensis	T	Pinaceae
HEMLOCK, Western	T. heterophylla	T	"
HEMP	Cannabis sativa	W	Cannabidaceae
HICKORY, Shagbark	Carya ovata	T	Jugulandaceae
HICKORY, Shellbark	C. laciniosa	T	"
HICKORY, White, (Mockernut)	C. tomentosa	T	"
HOPS, Cultivated	Humulus lupulus	W	Cannabidaceae
HOP-SAGE	Grayia spinosa	W	Chenopodiaceae
HORNBEAM, American	Carpinus carolineana	T	Carpinaceae
HORNBEAM, Hop, (Ironwood)	Ostrya virginiana	T	Carpinaceae
IODINE BUSH (Burroweed)	Allenrolfea occidentalis	W	Chenopodiaceae
JERUSALEM OAK	Chenopodium botrys	W	Chenopodiaceae
JOHNSONGRASS	Sorghum halepense	G	Gramineae
JUNIPER, California	Juniperus californica	T	Cupressaceae

Distribution	Pollination Period	Importance		
		Aller-genic	Plant	Pollen
Cultivated ornamental	Aug.-Sept.	B	B	B
MS. to AR. and TX.	July-Oct.	B	B	B
Cultivated ornamental	Mar.-Apr.	B	B	B
PQ. and ME. to ND., S. to FL. and TX.	Mar.-Arp.	B	B	B
Widespread weed	June-Aug.	C	B	C
AK. to S. CA., to ID. and MT.	Summer	C	B	C
NFLD. to SASK., S. to FL. and TX.	Summer	C	C	C
Cultivated forage and lawn grass	May-Aug.	A	A	A
AK. to NFLD., S. to S. CA., NM., TX., and SC.	June-Aug.	B	B	A
AK. to NFLD., S. to CA., NM., and NY.	May-Aug.	B	B	A
S.W. BC. to C. CA., E. to S.W. ALTA., MT., WY., CO., W. TX.	Apr.-May	C	B	C
Cascade Mts., WA., OR., CA.	June-July	C	B	C
W. WY., S. ID. to NM., AZ., CA.	May-June	C	B	C
Widespread weed, still advancing	Aug.-Oct.	A	A	A
Widespread weed	July-Sept.	C	C	C
S.E. US.	Summer-Fall	C	C	B
Widespread weed	May-Oct.	C	A	C
Widespread weed	Most of year esp. Srping	C	C	C
S. Canada to S. Mexico, E, to WI., IL., OK., W. to Mt., NV., S. CA.	Summer-Fall	C	B	C
S. CO. to E. WA., ALTA., ND., TX.	May-Aug.	B	B	B
Cultivated ornamental	Dec.-May	B	B	B
CT. to S. OH., S. IL., OK., S. to FL., TX., cultivated ornamental	May	C	B	C
PQ. to MAN., S. to NC., TN., AR.	Spring	B	B	B
ME. to SASK., S. to GA. and OK.	Jan.-Apr.	B	B	B
NFLD. to BC., S. to N. NJ., PA., OH., MO., N. GA. W. to N. CA., OR., WA.	Jan.-Apr.	B	B	B
NB. to ONT. and N. MN., S. to DE., WV., E. OH., C. MI., WI.	May-June	C	B	C
AK., to N. CA., to S.E. BC., N. ID., to N.W. MT.	May-June	C	B	C
Cultivated crop and widespread weed, diminishing	July-Sept.	C	C	B
PQ. and ME. to MI. and S.E. MN., S. FL. and TX.	May-June	B	B	B
NY. to S. ONT. to IA., S. to NC., MS., OK.	May-June	B	B	B
MA. to ONT., MI., IA., S. to FL. and TX.	May-June	B	B	B
Cultivated crop	Summer	C	C	B
CA. to E. WA., WY., AZ.	Mar.-June	C	C	B
NS. to MN., S. to FL. and TX.	Mar.-May	C	B	C
NS. to MAN., S. to FL. and TX.	Mar.-Apr.	C	B	C
CA. to OR., UT.	June-Aug.	B	B	B
Widespread weed	June-Oct.	B	B	B
Widespread weed over much of C. and S. US.	July-Oct.	B	A	B
C. and S. CA.	Jan.-Mar.	B	B	B

Name: Common	Name: Technical	Plant Form	Family
JUNIPER, Chinese	J. chinensis	T	,,
JUNIPER, Mountain	J. sabinoides	T	,,
JUNIPER, One-seed	J. monosperma	T	,,
JUNIPER, Pinchot	J. pinchotii	T	,,
JUNIPER, Rocky Mountain	J. scopulorum	T	,,
JUNIPER, Utah	J. utahensis	T	,,
JUNIPER, Virginia (Red Cedar)	Juniperus virginiana	T	,,
JUNIPER, Western	J. occidentalis	T	,,
KNOTGRASS	Paspalum distichum	G	Gramineae
KOELERGRASS (Junegrass)	Koeleria cristata	G	Gramineae
LARCH (Tamarack)	Larix occidentalis	T	Pinaceae
LENSCALE	Atriplex lentiformis	W	Chenopodiaceae
LINDEN, American	Tilia americana	T	Tiliaceae
LOCUST, Black	Robinia pseudoacacia	T	Leguminosae
MARSHELDER, August	Iva angustifolia	W	Compositae
MARSHELDER, Rough (Povertyweed)	I. ciliata	W	,,
MAPLE, Bigleaf (Canyon, Coast)	Acer macrophyllum	T	Aceraceae
MAPLE, Red	A. rubrum	T	,,
MAPLE, Silver (Soft Maple)	A. saccharinum	T	,,
MAPLE, Sugar	A. saccharum	T	,,
MELIC, California	Melica imperfecta	G	Gramineae
MESQUITE	Prosopis juliflora	T	Leguminosae
MOCK ORANGE (Syringa)	Philadelphus spp.	T	Philadelphaceae
MUGWORT	Artemisia douglasiana	W	Compositae
MUGWORT	A. heterophylla	W	,,
MULBERRY, Black	Morus tatarica	T	Moraceae
MULBERRY, Paper	Broussonetia papyrifera	T	Moraceae
MULBERRY, Red	Morus rubra	T	Moraceae
MULBERRY, White	M. alba	T	,,
MUSTARD, Black	Brassica nigra	W	Cruciferae
MUSTARD, Field (Common Ylw.)	B. campestris	W	,,
NETTLE	Urtica dioica	W	Urticaceae
OAK, Ariz. Scrub (Canyon Oak)	Quercus chrysolepsis	T	Fagaceae
OAK, Arizona White)	Q. arizonica	T	,,
OAK, Black	Q. velutina	T	,,
OAK, Black Jack	Q. marilandica	T	,,
OAK, Blue	Q. douglasii	T	,,
OAK, Bur	Q. macrocarpa	T	,,

Distribution	Pollination Period	Importance		
		Aller-genic	Plant	Pollen
Cultivated ornamental	Winter-Spring	C	C	B
W. and S. TX. into Mexico	Winter	B	B	B
N.W. OK., W. TX. to UT., NV., S.E. AZ., and NM.	Spring	B	B	B
C. TX. to S.E. NM., W. OK.	Spring	B	B	B
S. BC. to MT., ND., SD., Rocky Mountain States	May-June	B	B	B
CA. to S.W. ID., S.W. WY., W. NM.	Spring	B	B	B
S. PQ. and ME. to ND., S. to AL., TX.	Mar.-Apr.	B	B	B
Mountain slopes and higher. Prairies of E. WA., W. ID., S. in MT. Ranges to S. CA.	May-June	B	B	B
Common E. and S. US., occasional elsewhere	Aug.-Oct.	C	C	B
BC. to CA., E. to ONT. and ME., DE., LA., TX.	May-July	B	B	B
S. BC., S. to E. Cascades to OR., E. to N.W. MT., N, ID.	May-June	C	C	C
S. and C. CA. to UT.	Aug.-Oct.	A	A	A
PQ. to ND., S. to VA., NC., KY., MO.	June-July	C	B	C
PA. to S. IN. and OK., S. to GA., LA., cultivated ornamental	June	C	B	C
AR., OK., TX., LA.	Late Summer-Fall	B	B	B
IL. to LA., W. to NB., NM.	Late Spring-Summer	A	A	A
CA. to AK.	Apr.-May	C	B	C
PQ. to MN., S. to FL. and TX.	Mar.-Apr.	B	B	B
NB., PQ. to MN., SD., S. to FL., TN., OK., cultivated ornamental	Mar.-Apr.	B	B	B
PQ. and NJ. to MAN., ND., S. to NJ., GA., AL., TX.	Apr.-May	B	B	B
C. and S. CA.	Apr.-May	C	C	C
C. and S. CA. to Gulf of Mexico	Apr.-June	B	B	B
Cultivated ornamentals and widespread native shrubs	May-June	C	C	C
CA. E. to W. NV., to WA., ID.	June-Oct.	A	A	A
BC. to lower CA., SASK. to ID.	Summer	A	A	A
Cultivated ornamental	Spring	B	B	B
Cultivated ornamental	Winter-Spring	B	B	B
Cultivated ornamental	Spring	B	B	B
Cultivated ornamental	Spring	B	B	B
Widespread weed	Apr.-July	C	A	C
Widespread weed, especially in CA.	Jan.-May	C	A	C
Widespread weed	July-Sept.	B	B	B
S. CA. to OR., NM.	Apr.-May	B	B	B
W. TX. to AZ.	Spring	B	B	B
S. ME. to MI., MN., S. to FL. and TX.	Spring	B	B	B
S. NY. to S. MI., IA., S. to FL. and TX.	Spring	B	B	B
CA.	Apr.-May	B	B	B
NB., PQ. to ONT. and S. MAN., S. to VA., AL., AR., TX. Shrub in W. MN. and IA. to Canada	Spring	B	B	B

Name: Common	Name: Technical	Plant Form	Family
OAK, California Black	Q. kelloggii	T	"
OAK, California Scrub	Q. dumosa	T	"
OAK, Chestnut	Q. prinus	T	"
OAK, Coast Live (Encina)	Q. agrifolia	T	"
OAK, Emory	Q. emoryi	T	Fagaceae
OAK, Engelmann	Q. engelmannii	T	"
OAK, Gambel	Q. gambelii	T	"
OAK, Garry	Q. garryana	T	"
OAK, Holly	Q. ilex	T	"
OAK, Interior Live	Q. wislizenii	T	"
OAK, Palmer	Q. palmeri	T	"
OAK, Pin	Q. palustris	T	"
OAK, Post	Quercus stellata	T	"
OAK, Red (Northern Red Oak)	Q. rubra (Q. borealis)	T	"
OAK, Spanish (Southern Red Oak)	Q. falcata	T	"
OAK, Valley (Roble)	Q. lobata	T	"
OAK, Virginia Live	Q. virginiana	T	"
OAK, Water	Q. nigra	T	"
OAK, White	Q. alba	T	"
OATGRASS, Tall	Arrhenatherum elatius	G	Gramineae
OATS, Common Wild	Avena fatua	G	Gramineae
OATS, Cultivated	A. sativa	G	"
OATS, Slender Wild	A. barbata	G	"
OLIVE	Olea europaea	T	Oleaceae
ORANGE, Osage	Maclura pomifera	T	Moraceae
ORCHARDGRASS	Dactylis glomerata	G	Gramineae
PALM, Canary Island Date	Phoenix canariensis	T	Palmae
PALM, Date	P. dactylifera	T	"
PALM, Dwarf	Chamaerops humilis	T	Palmae
PALM, Queen	Cocos plumosa	T	Palmae
PALO VERDE	Cercidium torreyana	T	Leguminosae
PAMPASGRASS	Cortaderia selloana	G	Gramineae
PEA, Sweet	Lathyrus odoratus	W	Leguminosae
PEACH	Prunus persica	T	Rosaceae
PEAR	Pyrus communis	T	Rosaceae
PECAN	Carya pecan	T	Juglandaceae
PEPPERTREE, Brazilian	Schinus terebinthifolius	T	Anacardiaceae
PEPPERTREE, Peruvian	S. molle	T	"
PHLOX	Phlox spp.	W	Polemoniaceae
PICKLEWEED (Glasswort)	Salicornia ambigua	W	Chenopodiaceae

Distribution	Pollination Period	Importance		
		Allergenic	Plant	Pollen
S. CA. to OR.	Apr.-May	B	B	B
CA.	Mar.-May	B	B	B
Appalachian Mts., ME. to N. GA. to Atlantic Coast as far as S. VA., W. to S. IN.	Spring	B	B	B
C. and S. CA.	Mar.-Apr.	A	A	A
TX. to AZ.	Spring	B	B	B
S. CA.	Apr.-May	B	B	B
S.W. TX. to CO., WY., S. to AZ., abundant on dry slopes of Rockies	Spring	B	B	B
N. CA., W. OR., WA.	Spring	A	A	A
Cultivated ornamental	Spring	C	C	C
C. and N. CA.	Mar.-May	B	B	B
S. CA., AZ.	Apr.-May	B	B	B
MA. to MI., IA., E. KS., S. to NC., TN., OK.	Spring	B	B	B
S.E. MA., S. NY. to OH., IN., IA., S. to FL. and TX.	Spring	B	B	B
NS. to N. MI. and MN., S. to VA., AL., MS., AR.	Spring	B	B	B
NJ., PA. to FL. and TX., along coastal plain and N. in interior to OH., IN., MD.	Spring	B	B	B
C. and S. CA.	Mar.-Apr.	B	B	B
Coastal plain, S.E. VA. to FL. and TX.	Spring	B	B	B
Coastal plain, DE. to FL. and S.E. TX., N. in interior to S.E. MO.	Spring	B	B	B
ME. to MI. and MN., S. to FL. and TX.	Spring	B	B	B
S.W. BC. to CA. E. across Canada to ID. and MT.	May-July	B	B	B
Common throughout W. North America	Mar.-Sept.	B	B	B
Cultivated crop	May-Aug.	C	C	C
S.W. US.	May-June	C	C	C
Cultivated crop and ornamental	May-June	B	B	B
Cultivated hedge and native tree, AR., OK., TX.	Apr.-May	C	B	C
Common throughout most of North America	June-Aug.	A	A	A
Cultivated ornamental	Spring	C	C	C
Cultivated crop and ornamental	Spring	C	C	C
Cultivated ornamental	Spring	C	C	C
Cultivated ornamental	Spring	C	C	C
S. CA., AZ.	Mar.-May	C	c	C
Cultivated ornamental	June-Sept.	C	C	C
Cultivated ornamental	Jan.-Dec.	C	C	C
Cultivated crop and ornamental	Mar.-May	C	C	C
Cultivated crop	Mar.-May	C	C	C
Cultivated crop and ornamental, S.W. OH. to IA., S. to AL., TX.	Spring	B	B	B
Cultivated ornamental naturalized in S. FL.	Jan.-Dec.	C	C	C
Cultivated ornamental	Winter	C	C	C
Cultivated ornamental	Spring-Summer	C	C	C
Atlantic and Pacific coastal, salt marshes and adjacent salt flats	Aug.-Nov.	C	B	C

Name: Common	Name: Technical	Plant Form	Family
PIGWEED, Green	Amaranthus hybridus	W	Amaranthaceae
PIGWEED, Redroot	A. retroflexus	W	"
PIGWEED, Spiny	A. spinosus	W	"
PIGWEED, Spreading	A. blitoides	W	"
PINE, AUSTRAL.: see Beefwood	Casuarina equisetifolia	T	Casuarinaceae
PINE, Bull (Digger)	Pinus sabiniana	T	Pinaceae
PINE, Canary Island	P. canariensis	T	"
PINE, Eastern White	P. strobus	T	"
PINE, Japanese Black	P. thunbergii	T	"
PINE, Loblolly	P. taeda	T	"
PINE, Lodgepole	P. contorta	T	"
PINE, Longleaf	P. palustris (P. australis)	T	"
PINE, Monterey	P. radiata	T	"
PINE, Pinyon	P. edulis	T	"
PINE, Ponderosa (West. Yellow)	P. ponderosa	T	"
PINE, Red (Norway)	P. resinosa	T	"
PINE, Short-leaf (Yellow)	P. echinata	T	Pinaceae
PINE, Single-leaf (One-leaved)	P. monophylla	T	"
PINE, Virginia Scrub (Jersey)	P. virginiana	T	"
PINE, Western White	P. monticola	T	"
PLANTAIN, Common	Plantago major	W	Plantaginaceae
PLANTAIN, English (Buckhorn)	P. lanceolata	W	"
PLUM	Prunus domestica	T	Rosaceae
POPLAR, Balsam	Populus balsamifera	T	Salicaceae
POPLAR, Black	P. nigra	T	"
POPLAR, Lombardy	P. nigra italica	T	"
POPLAR, White (Silver)	P. alba	T	"
POPPY, California	Escholtzia californica	W	Papaveraceae
POVERTYWEED, Small	Iva axillaris	W	Compositae
POVERTYWEED, Giant	I. xanthifolia	W	"
PRIVET, California	Ligustrum ovalifolium	T	Oleaceae
PRIVET, Common	L. vulgare	T	"
PRIVET, Southern	L. lucidum	T	"
QUACKGRASS	Agropyron repens	G	Gramineae
LAMBSQUARTERS (Pigweed)	Chenopodium album	W	Chenopodiaceae
RABBITBRUSH	Chrysothamnus nauseosus	W	Compositae
RABBITBUSH	Franseria deltoides	W	Compositae
RAGWEED, Canyon	F. ambrosioides	W	"
RAGWEED, Desert (Burroweed)	F. dumosa	W	"
RAGWEED, False, (Sandbur)	F. acanthicarpa	W	"
RAGWEED, Giant (Crownweed)	Ambrosia trifida	W	Compositae

Distribution	Pollination Period	Importance		
		Allergenic	Plant	Pollen
Widespread weed	June-Nov.	B	B	B
Widespread weed	June-Nov.	A	A	A
Advancing weed	June-Sept.	B	B	B
Widespread weed	July-Nov.	B	B	B
Cultivated ornamental	Spring	C	C	C
C. and S. CA.	Apr.-May	C	B	C
Cultivated ornamental	Spring	C	C	C
NFLD. to MAN., S. to DE., GA., KY., IA.	Spring	C	B	C
Cultivated ornamental	Spring	C	C	C
NJ. to FL., TX., N. in interior to AR. and TN.	Spring	C	B	C
CA., AK., Rocky Mts.	June-July	C	B	C
Coastal plain, S.E. VA. to FL. and TX.	Spring	C	B	C
Monterey Peninsula and adjacent coastal counties	Apr.	C	B	C
S. CA. to WY., TX., AZ.	Spring	C	B	C
S. CA. to BC., Rocky Mts.	May-June	C	B	C
NS. to MAN., S. to MA., PA., MI., MN., in mts. to WV.	Spring	C	B	C
S. NY. to WV., S. IL., S.E. KS., S. to FL. and TX.	Spring	C	B	C
C. and E. CA. to UT., AZ.	May	C	B	C
S. NY. to S. IN., S. to GA., AL.	Spring	C	B	C
S. BC. to CA., W. NV., E. to ID., S.W. AK., W. MT.	May-June	C	B	C.
Widespread weed	Jan.-Dec.	C	A	C
Widespread weed	June-Sept.	A	A	A
Cultivated crop and ornamental	Mar.-May	C	C	C
LAB. to AK., S. to CT., N. PA., N. IN., IA., NB., OR.	Mar.-Apr.	B	B	B
Cultivated ornamental	Mar.-Apr.	C	C	B
Cultivated ornamental	Mar.-Apr.	C	C	B
Cultivated ornamental	Mar.-Apr.	C	C	B
CA., cultivated ornamental elsewhere	Feb.-Sept.	C	C	C
CA. to NB., Canada	May-Sept.	B	B	B
PQ. to ALTA., S. to DC., OH., MD., TX., NM., AZ.	July-Sept.	B	B	B
Cultivated ornamental	Spring	C	C	C
Cultivated ornamental	Spring-Summer	C	C	C
Cultivated ornamental	Spring	C	C	C
Widespread in much of temperate and sub-arctic North America, except deserts	June-Aug.	B	A	B
Widespread weed	June-Oct.	A	A	A
E. CA., N. to BC., E. to SASK., TX.	July-Oct.	C	B	C
S. AZ. and Mexico	Spring	A	B	A
S. CA., S. AZ.	Mar.-June	A	B	A
S. CA., S.W. UT., AZ.	Mar.-May	A	A	A
C. and S. CA. to WA., SASK., TX, advancing eastward	Aug.-Nov.	A	A	A
S. Canada and US. to Rocky Mts.	July-Sept.	A	A	A

Name: Common	Name: Technical	Plant Form	Family
RAGWEED, Short	A. artemisifolia	W	,,
RAGWEED, Silver	Dicoria canescens	W	Compositae
RAGWEED, Slender	Franseria tenuifolia	W	Compositae
RAGWEED, Southern	Ambrosia bidentata	W	Compositae
RAGWEED, Western	A. psilostachya	W	,,
REDSCALE	Atriplex rosea	W	Chenopodiaceae
REDTOP	Agrostis alba	G	Gramineae
REDWOOD	Sequoia sempervirens	T	Taxodiaceae
RESCUEGRASS (South. Chess)	Bromus uniloides (cathariticus)	G	Gramineae
RIPGUT	B. rigidus	G	,,
ROSE	Rosa spp.	W	Rosaceae
RYE, Cultivated	Secale cerale	G	Gramineae
RYEGRASS, Alkali	Elymus triticoides	G	Gramineae
RYEGRASS, Giant	E. condensatus	G	,,
RYEGRASS, Italian (Annual)	Lolium multiflorum	G	Gramineae
RYEGRASS, Perennial	L. perenne	G	,,
RYEGRASS, Western	Elymus glaucus	G	Gramineae
SAGEBRUSH, Annual	Artemisia annua	W	Compositae
SAGEBRUSH, Biennial	A. biennis	W	,,
SAGEBRUSH, California	A. californica	W	,,
SAGEBRUSH, Carpet (Pasture)	A. frigida	W	,,
SAGEBRUSH, Common (Giant)	A. tridentata	W	,,
SAGEBRUSH, Prairie	A. ludoviciana	W	,,
SAGEBRUSH, Sand Dune	A. pycnocephala	W	,,
SAGEBRUSH, Suksdorf	A. suksdorfii	W	,,
SALTBUSH, Annual	Atriplex wrightii	W	Chenopodiaceae
SALTGRASS, Coastal	Distichlis spicata	G	Gramineae
SALTGRASS, Desert	D. stricta	G	,,
SEDGE	Carex spp.	W	Cyperaceae
SHADSCALE (Sheep Fat)	Atriplex conifertifolia	W	Chenopodiaceae
SEA BLITE (Seepweed)	Suaeda moquini	W	Chenopodiaceae
SEA BLITE (Seepweed)	S. californica	W	,,
SEA BLITE (Seepweed)	S. suffrutescens	W	,,
SHEEP SORREL	Rumex acetosella	W	Polygonaceae
SILK TASSEL BUSH	Garrya elliptica	T	Garryaceae
SILVERSCALE	Atriplex argentea	W	Chenopodiaceae
SNAPDRAGON	Antirrhinum majus	W	Scrophulariaceae
SORGHUM	Sorghum vulgare	G	Gramineae
SPEARSCALE	Atriplex patula	W	Chenopodiaceae
SPIRAEA (Bridal Wreath)	Spiraea spp.	T	Rosaceae
SPRUCE, Colorado Blue	Picea pungens	T	Pinaceae
SPRUCE, Red	P. rubens	T	,,

Distribution	Pollination Period	Importance		
		Allergenic	Plant	Pollen
S. Canada and US., except W. and S.W. US.	Aug.-Oct.	A	A	A
S. CA., S.W. AZ., NV., S.W. UT.	Sept.-Jan.	B	B	A
C. and S. CA. to KS., TX.	May-Nov.	B	B	A
S. IL. to LA., W. to NB. and TX.	Aug.-Sept.	B	B	A
CA. to WA., SASK., IL.	July-Nov.	A	A	A
CA. to WA., Atlantic Coast	July-Oct.	B	B	B
Widespread in Canada and US.	June-Sept.	A	A	A
C. CA. to S.W. OR.	Mar.	C	C	C
Cultivated for forage in S. states	Summer	B	B	B
BC. to S. CA., E. to ID., Rocky Mts. in CO. and NM.	Apr.-June	B	A	B
Cultivated ornamentals and native shrubs	Jan.-Dec.	C	B	C
Cultivated crop	May-July	C	C	B
C. WA. to S. CA., E. to MT., WY., CO., NM.	June-Aug.	B	B	B
CA.	June-Aug.	B	B	B
Cultivated lawn grass and widespread weed	May-July	A	A	A
Cultivated forage crop and lawn grass	May-July	A	A	A
S. AK. to S. CA., E. to ONT., MI., IN., IA., CO., NM.	June-Aug.	B	B	B
Widespread weed	July-Sept.	C	C	B
Widespread weed	Aug.-Sept.	C	C	B
Coastal C. and S. CA.	Aug.-Dec.	A	A	A
Some forms cultivated annuals	July-Sept.	A	A	A
S. CA. to BC., Rocky Mts.	Aug.-Oct.	A	A	A
CA. to WA., ALTA., ONT., AR., NM.	July-Sept.	A	A	A
Coastal C. CA. and OR.	June-Aug.	B	B	B
Coastal N. CA. to Vancouver Island	May-Aug.	B	B	B
S. AZ. and S. NM.	July-Sept.	B	B	B
Vancouver Island to S. CA., Canada to FL., LA., TX.	June-Sept.	B	B	B
S. BC. to S. CA., E. to SASK., MO., OK., TX.	May-July	B	B	B
Widespread, largest genus of flowering plants in North America	Spring-Summer	C	A	C
S. CA. to E. OR., ND.	Apr.-July	B	B	B
S. CA. to ALTA.	July-Oct.	B	B	B
Coastal salt marsh, San Francisco Bay to S. CA.	July-Oct.	B	B	B
C. CA. to WA., Rocky Mts.	July-Sept.	B	B	B
Widespread weed	Mar.-Aug.	A	A	A
C. CA. to OR.	Jan.-Mar.	C	C	C
S. CA. to BC., ND., NM.	June-Sept.	B	B	B
Cultivated crop	Jan.-Dec.	C	C	C
Cultivated crop	Jan.-Dec.	C	C	C
Widespread weed	June-Nov.	B	B	B
Cultivated ornamentals and widespread native shrubs	Spring-Summer	C	C	C
Cultivated ornamental, native to C. CO.	June-July	C	C	C
PQ. and ONT. to PA., NJ., S. in mts. to NC. and TN.	Spring-Summer	C	B	C

Name: Common	Name: Technical	Plant Form	Family
SPRUCE, Sitka	P. sitchensis	T	"
SUDANGRASS	Sorghum sudanense	G	Gramineae
SUNFLOWER	Helianthus spp.	W	Compositae
SWEET GALE	Myrica gale	T	Myricaceae
SYCAMORE (London Plane)	Platanus orientalis	T	Platanaceae
SYCAMORE, Eastern (Buttonwood)	P. occidentalis	T	"
SYCAMORE, Maple-leaf	P. acerifolia	T	"
SYCAMORE, Western	P. racemosa	T	"
TANSY	Tanacetum vulgare	W	Compositae
TARRAGON (Green Sagebrush)	Artemisia dracunculus	W	Compositae
TARWEED	Hemizonia spp.	W	Compositae
TEA, Mexican (Wormseed)	Chenopodium ambrosioides	W	Chenopodiaceae
THISTLE, Russian	Salsola kali	W	Chenopodiaceae
TIMOTHY	Phleum pratense	G	Gramineae
TREE-OF-HEAVEN	Ailanthus altissima	T	Simaroubaceae
TULIP	Tulipa spp.	W	Liliaceae
VERNALGRASS, Sweet	Anthoxanthum odoratum	G	Gramineae
VELVETGRASS	Holcus lanatus	G	Gramineae
VIBURNUM	Viburnum spp.	T	Caprifoliaceae
WALNUT, Arizona	Juglans rupestris	T	Juglandaceae
WALNUT, Black	J. nigra	T	"
WALNUT, California Black	J. californica	T	"
WALNUT, English	J. regia	T	"
WALNUT, Hinds' Black	J. hindsii	T	"
WALNUT, Japanese	J. sieboldiana	T	"
WATERHEMP	Acnida tamariscina	W	Amaranthaceae
WHEAT, Cultivated	Triticum aestivum	G	Gramineae
WHEATGRASS, Crested	Agropyron cristatum	G	Gramineae
WHEATGRASS, Slender	A. tenerum	G	"
WHEATGRASS, Western	A. smithii	G	"
WILLOW, Arroyo	Salix lasiolepis	T	Salicaceae
WILLOW, Black	S. nigra	T	"
WILLOW, Pussy	S. discolor	T	"
WILLOW, Red	S. laevigata	T	"
WILLOW, Yellow	S. lasiandra	T	"
WINGSCALE (Shadscale)	Atriplex canescens	W	Chenopodiaceae
WINTER FAT	Eurotia lanata	W	Chenopodiaceae
WORMWOOD	Artemisia absinthium	W	Compositae

Distribution	Pollination Period	Importance		
		Aller-genic	Plant	Pollen
AK. to C. CA. in Coastal Mts.	May	C	B	C
Cultivated crop	Jan.-Dec.	C	C	C
Cultivated crop, ornamental, native S. Canada to Mexican border	Feb.-Oct.	C	B	C
Circumboreal, in North America, S. to NY., PA., NC., MI., MN., WA.	Apr.-June	C	C	C
Cultivated ornamental	Spring	C	C	B
S.W. ME. to S. MI. and S.E. MN., S. to FL., TX.	Spring	B	B	B
Cultivated ornamental	Spring	B	B	B
C. and S. CA.	Feb.-Apr.	B	B	B
Cultivated ornamental, naturalized weed	July-Sept.	C	B	C
C. and S. CA., N. to BC., WI., TX, cultivated form sterile	Aug.-Oct.	B	B	B
30+ spp., all in CA.	Apr.-Nov.	C	C	C
Widespread weed	June-Dec.	B	B	B
Widespread weed	July-Oct.	A	A	A
Cultivated hay crop	June-Aug.	A	A	A
Cultivated ornamental and urban weed	June	C	C	C
Cultivated ornamentals	Spring	C	C	C
AK., BC. to CA., E. Canada, C. and E. US.	Apr.-July	A	A	A
AK. to CA., E. to NFLD., S. to GA., TN., MO., AZ., except Rocky Mts.	July-Sept.	A	A	A
Cultivated ornamental, widespread native shrubs	May-July	C	C	C
W. OK., TX. to S.E. NM., AZ.	Spring	B	B	B
Cultivated crop, ornamental native W. New England to MI., MN., NB., S. to FL. TX.	Apr.-May	B	B	B
S. CA.	Apr.-May	B	B	B
Cultivated crop	Apr.-May	B	B	B
C. and N. CA.	Apr.-May	B	B	B
Cultivated ornamental	Apr.-May	C	C	B
E. TX., N. to S. OK., E. to IN.	Aug.-Sept.	A	A	A
Cultivated crop	Apr.-June	C	B	C
Arid W. US.	June-Aug.	A	A	A
AK. to S. CA., Pacific to Atlantic Coast	June-Aug.	A	A	A
BC. S. to E. WA., OR., NV., AZ., E. to ONT., NY., TN., TX.	June-Aug.	A	A	A
CA. to WA., ID., NM.	Feb.-Apr.	C	B	C
S. NB. to C. MN., S. to FL., TX.	Spring	C	B	C
Cultivated ornamental, native shrub, NFLD. to BC., S. to DE., KY., MO., SD., MT.	Spring	C	B	C
CA., UT., AZ.	Mar.-May	C	B	C
CA. to AK., ID.	Mar.-May	C	B	C
C. and S. CA. to E. WA., SD., KS., TX.	June-Aug.	A	A	A
C. and S. CO., WA., Rocky Mts., TX.	Mar.-June	B	B	B
Cultivated ornamental, naturalized weed	July-Sept.	B	B	B

✦ BIBLIOGRAPHY

GENERAL INFORMATION:

1 • Korenblat, Phillip E., M.D.: Allergy: Theory and Practice, Grune & Stratton, Inc.

2 • Slavin, Raymond G.: The Allergy Encyclopedia, New American Library, New York.

3 • Speer, Frederic: Handbook of clinical allergy: A Practical Guide to Patient Management. Boston, John Wright, PSG Inc., 1982.

4 • Swinny, B., in Speer, F: "The Allergic Child." New York, Harper and Row, 1963.

ALLERGENS:

DUST

1 • Baker, E.W., Evans, T.M. Gould, D.J. "A manual of parasitic mites of medical or economic importance." New York: National Pest Control Association, Inc., 1956.

2 • Arlian, L.G., Gernstein, I.L., and Gallagher, J.S.: The prevalence of house dust mites Dermatophagoides and associate environmental conditions in homes in Ohio, J. Allergy Clin. Immunol. 69:527, 1982.

3 • Bagenstose, A.H., Mathews, K.P., Homburger, H.A., and Saavedra-Delgado, A.P.: Inhalant allergy due to crickets J. Allergy Clin. Immunol. 65:71, 1980.

4 • Bernecker, C.: Mites and house dust allergy, Lancet 2:1145, 1968.

5 • Bernton, H.S., McMahon, T.F., and Brown, H.: Cockroach asthma, Br. J.Dis. Chest 66:61, 1972.

6 • Berrens, L.: Kapok allergens, Int. Arch. Allergy Appl. Immunol. 29:575, 1966.

7 • Berrens, L.: On the composition of feather extracts used in allergy practice, Int. Arch. Allergy App. Immunol. 34:81, 1968.

8 • Berrens, L.: Structural studies of house dust allergens. Clin. Exp. Immunol. 6:71, 1970.

9 • Berrens, L.: The allergens in house dust, Prog. Allergy 14:259, 1970.

10 • Berrens, L.: On the composition of feather extracts used in allergy practice. Int. Arch. Allergy Appl. Immunol. 1968, 34, 81.

11 • Clark, R. P., Preston, T.D., Gordon-Nesbitt, C.D., et al.: The size of airborne dust particles precipitating bronchospasm in house dust sensitive children, J. Hygiene 77:321, 1976.

12 • Cohen, M.B., Nelson, T., and Reinarz, B.H.: Observations on the nature of the house dust allergy, J. Allergy 6:517, 1935.

13 • Collins-Williams, C., Hung. F., and Bremner, K.: House dust mite and house dust allergy, Ann. Allergy 37:12, 1976.

14 • Hughes, A., Maunsell, K.: A study of a population of house dust mite in its natural environment, Clinical Allergy, 3:127-131.

15 • Kawai, T., Marsh, D.G., Lichtenstein, L.M., and Norman, P.S.: The allergens responsible for house dust allergy. 1. Comparison of "Dermatophagoides pteronyssinus" and house dust extracts by assay of histamine release from allergic human leukocytes, J. Allergy Clin. Immunol. 50:117, 1972.

16 • Korgaard, J.: Preventive measures in house dust allergy, Am. Rev. Respir. Dis. 1251:80, 1982.

17 • Le Mao, J., Sandell, J.P., Rabillion, J., et al.: Antigens and allergens in "Dematophagoides farinae" mite, Immunology 44:239, 1981.

18 • Lind, P., Korsgaard, J., and Lowenstein, H. Detection and quantitation of "Dermatophagoides" antigens in house dust by immunochemical techniques, Allergy 34:319, 1979.

19 • Miyamoto, T., Oshima, S., Ishizaki, T., and Sato, S.: Allergenic identity between the common floor mite ("Dermatophagoides farinae" Hughes, 1961) and house dust as a causative antigen in bronchial asthma, J. Allergy 42:14, 1968.

20 • Miyamoto, T., Oshima, S., and Ishizaki, T.: Antigenic relation between house dust and dust mite ("Dermatophagoides farinae" Hughes, 1961) by a fractionation method, J. Allergy 44:282, 1969.

21 • Morita, Y., Miyamoto, T., Horinchi, Y., et al.: Further studies in allergic identity between house dust and the house dust mite,("Detmatophagoides farinae" Hughes, 1961), Ann. Allergy 35:361, 1975.

22 • Mulla, M., Harkrider, J., Galant, S., Amin, L.: Some house-dust control measures and abundance of "Dermatophagoides" mites in Southern California, J. Med. Ent. 12:5, 1975.

23 • Murray, A., Ferguson, A.: Dust-free bedrooms in the treatment of asthmatic children with house dust or house dust mite allergy: A controlled trial.

24 • Murray, A., and Zuk, P.: The seasonal variation in a population of house dust mites in a North American city, J. Allergy Clin. Immunol. 64:266, 1979.

25 • Rao, V., Dean, B., Seaton, A., Williams, D.: A comparison of mite populations in mattress dust from hospital and from private houses in Cardiff, Wales, Clinical Allergy, 5:209, 1975.

26 • Sarfield,J.K.: Role of house-dust mites in childhood asthma, Arch. Dis. Child, 49:711, 1974.

27 • Sarfield, J.K., Gowland, G., Toy, R., and Norman, A.L.: Mite-sensitive asthma of childhood: trial of avoidance measures, Arch. Dis. Child. 49:716, 1974.

28 • Torey, E.R., Chapman, M.D., Wells, C.W., and Platts-Mills, T.A.E.: The distribution of dust mite allergen in the houses of patients with asthma, Am. Rev. Respir. Dis. 124:630, 1981.

29 • Tovey, E.R., Chapman, M.D., Platts-Mills, T.A.E.: Mite faeces are a major source of house dust allergens, Nature 289:592, 1981.

30 • Voorhorst, R.: To what extent are house-dust mites ("Dermatophagoides") responsible for complaints in asthma patients? Allergy Immunol. 18:9, 1972.

31 • Voorhorst, R., Spieksma, F.T.M., Varekamp, H., et al.: The housedust mite (Dermatophagoides pteronyssinus) and the allergens it produces: identity with the house-dust allergen, J. Allergy 39:325, 1967.

32 • Warner, J.O., and Price, J.F.: Housedust mite sensitivity in childhood asthma, Arch. Dis. Child. 53:710, 1978.

POLLEN & MOLDS:

1 • Adams, D.E., Perkins, W.E., & Estes, J.R.: Am. J. Botl, 68:389, 1981.

2 • Dalen, G. Van, & Voorhorst, R.: Ann. Allergy, 46:276, 1981.

3 • Derbes, V.J.: J. Allergy, 12:502, 1941.

4 • Holopainen, E, Salo, O.P., Tarkiainen E, et al: The most important allergens in allergic rhinitis, Acta Otolaryngol (supp) 360:16, 1979.

5 • Lewis, W.H., & Imber, W.E.: Ann. Allergy, 35:42, 1975.

6 • Lewis, W.H., & Vinay, P.: Ann. Allegy, 42:309, 1979.

7 • Lewis, W.H., Vinay, P., & Zenger, V.E.: In airborne and allergenic pollen of North America.

8 • Michel, F.B., Cour, P., Quet, L., et al: Qualitative and quantitative comparison of pollen calendars for plain and mountain areas, Clin. Allergy, 6:383, 1976.

9 • Samter, M., Durham, O.C.: Regional allergy of the United States, Canada, Mexico, and Cuba, Springfield, Ill, Charles C. Thomas, 1955.

10 • Morrow, M.B., Meyer, G.H., Prince, H.E.: A summary of air-borne mold survey, Ann. Allergy 22:575, 1964.

11 • Dworin, M.: A study of atmospheric mold spores in Tucson, Arizona, Ann. Allergy 24:31, 1966.

12 • Sneller, M.R., Hayes, H.D., Pinnas, J.L.: Frequency of air-borne Alternaria spores in Tucson, Arizona, over a 20-year period, Ann. Allergy 46:30, 1981.

13 • Shapiro, R.S., Eisenberg, B.C., Binder, W.: The importance of field studies and meterologic factors in pollen and mold surveys, Ann. Allergy 46:484,1965.

14 • Seller, M.R., Roby, R.R.: Incidence of fungal spores at the homes of allergic patients in an agricultural community. I.A 12 month study in and out of doors, Ann. Allergy 23:484, 1965.

15 • Street, D.H., Hamburger, R.N.: Atmospheric pollen and spore sampling in San Diego, California. I. Meteorological correlations and potential clinical relevance, Ann. Allergy 37:32, 1976.

16 • Newmark, F.M.: The hay fever plants of Colorado, Ann. Allergy 40:18, 1978.

17 • Al-Doory, Y., Domson, J.E., Howard, W.C., et al: Airborne fungi and pollens of the Washington, D.C. metropolitan area, Ann. Allergy 45:360, 1980.

18 • Finegold, I.: A two-year pollen and spore survey of southeast Florida, Ann. Allergy 35:37, 1975.

19 • Sorenson, W.G., Bulmer, G.S, Criep, L.H.: Airborne fungi from five sites in the continental United States and Puerto Rico, Ann. Allergy 33:131, 1974.

20 • Roth, A., Shira, J.: Allergy in Hawaii, Ann. Allergy 24:73, 1966.

21 • McDevitt, T.J., Mallea, M., Dominick, T., et al: Allergic evaluation of cereal smuts, Ann. Allergy 38:12, 1977.

22 • Salvaggio, J., Zaslow, L, Greer, J., et al: New Orleans asthma. III. Semi-quantitative aerometric pollen sampling, 1967 and 1968. Ann. Allergy 29:305, 1971.

23 • Leventin, E., Buck, P.: Hay fever plants in Oklahoma. Ann. Allergy 45:26, 1980.

24 • Leventin, E., Horowitz, L.: A one-year survey of the airborne molds of Tulsa, Oklahoma. I. Outdoor survey. Ann. Allergy 41:21, 1978.

25 • Acosta, F., Roberstad, G.W.: Chrysosporium species as fungal air pollutants. Ann. Allergy 42:11, 1979.

26 • Anderson, E.F., Dorsett, C.S., Fleming, E.O.: The airborne pollens of Walla Walla, Washington. Ann. Allergy 41:21, 1978.

27 • Durham, O.C., Fafalla, H.: A pollen survey of the National Park and St. John's Island, Virgin Islands. J. Allergy 32:27, 1961.

28 • Bassett, I.J., Crompton, C.W., Parmelee, J.A.: "An Atlas of Airborne Pollen Grains and Common Fungus Spores of Canada." Quebec, Canada, Research Branch, Canada Department of Agriculture, 1978.

INSECTS:

1 • American Academy of Allergy, Insect Allergy Committee, 1963, report: J. Allergy 35:1181, 1964.

2 • Barr, S.E.: Immunotherapy in hypersensitivity to insects. (Letter) N. Engl. J. Med. 299:1135-1136, 1978.

3 • Busse, W.W., Reed, C.E., Lichtenstein, L.M., et al: Immunotherapy in bee sting anaphylaxia. JAMA 231:1154-115,1975.

4 • Feinberg, A.R., Feinberg, S.M. and Beniam-Pinto, C.: Asthma and rhinitis from insect allergens. I. Clinical importance. J. Allergy 27:437, 1956.

5 • Figley, K.D.: Asthma due to May fly. Am. J. Med. Sci. 178:338, 1929.

6 • Frazier, C.A.: Allergic reaction to insect stings. South Med. J. 57:1028-1034, 1964.

7 • Frazier, C.A.: Insect Allergy. St. Louis, Warren H. Green, 1969.

8 • Kern, R.A.: Asthma due to sensitivity to mushroom fly (*Aphiochaeti agarici*), J. Allergy 9:604, 1938.

9 • Lichtenstein, L.M., Valentine, M.D., Sobotka, A.K.J: Insect allergy: State of the art. J. Allergy Clin. Immunol 64:5-12, 1979.

10 • Mueller, H.L.: Maintenance of Protection in patients treated for stinging insect hypersensitivity. Pediatrics 59:773-776, 1977.

11 • Reisman, R.E.: Stinging insect allergy. J. Allergy Clin. Immunol 64:3-4, 1979.

12 • Rynes, S.E.: A critical analysis of animal dander reactions. J. Allergy 8:470, 1937.

13 • Way, K.D.: Water flea sensitivity, case report. J. Allergy 12:495, 1940.

14 • Wiseman, R.D., Woodin, R.L., Miller, H.C. and Myers, M.A.: Insect allergy as a possible cause of inhalant sensitivity. J. Allergy 30:191, 1959.

INDOOR AIR POLLUTION:

1 • Ashrae Standard. "Ventilation for Acceptable Indoor Air Quality." American Society of Heating Refrigeration and Air Conditioning Engineers. New York. 1980.

2 • Ban of urea-formaldehyde foam insulation, withdrawal of proposed information labeling rule, and denial of petition to issue a standard. Federal Register, Consumer Product Safety Commission. 47(67):14366-14421, 1982.

3 • Barbana, E.J.: Formaldehyde: hypersensitivity and irritant reactions at work and in the home. Immunol. Allergy Pract. 2:60-72, 1980.

4 • Bonin, J.: Shell Answer Book x The Chemical Do's and Dont's Book. Shell Oil Company. Houston, Texas, 1979.

5 • Breysse, P.A.: The health cost of tight homes. JAMA 245:267-268, 1981.

6 • Center for Science in the Public Interest. The Household Pollutants Guide. Anchor Press, New York, 1978.

7 • Consumer Research Magazine. "Dryer Fabric Softeners," 57, October, 1974.

8 • Consumer Research Magazine. "Enzyme Pre-soaks, Enzyme Detergents, and Soaps," 56. August, 1973.

9 • Dadashan, A.M.: The role of fiberglass dust in the origin of bronchial asthma. (Translation) Vrachenoe Delo 10:87, 1969.

10 • Dally, K.A., Hanrahan, M.A., Woodbury, M.A., Kanarek, M.A.: Formaldehyde exposure in non-occupational environments. Arch. Environ. Health 36:277-289, 1981.

11 • Day, J.H., Lees, R.E.M, Clarke, R.H.: Respiratory effects of formaldehyde and UFFI off-gas following controlled exposure. J. Allergy Clin. Immunol. 7:159, 1983 (suppl).

12 • Finnegan, M.J., Pickering, C.A.C., Burge, P.S.: "The sick building syndrome: prevalence studies." British Medical Journal, 289:1573, 1984.

13 • Fischer, M.H. "The toxic effects of formaldehyde and formalin." J Exp Med 6:487-518, 1905.

14 • Frigas, E., Filley, W.V., Reed, C.E.: Asthma induced by dust from urea-formaldehyde foam insulating material. Chest 79:706-707, 1981.

15 • Frigas, E., Filley, W.V., Redd, C.E.: UFFI dust. Non-specific irritant only? Chest 82:511-512, 1982.

16 • Garry, V.F., Oatman, L, Pleus, R., Gray, D.: Formaldehyde in the home. Some environmental disease perspectives. Minn. Med. 63:107, 1980.

17 • Godish, T.: Formaldehyde and building-related illness. J. Environ Health 44:116, 1981.

18 • Gupta, K.C., Ulsamer, A.G., Preuss, P.W.: Formaldehyde in indoor air: Sources and toxicity. International Symposium on Indoor Air Pollution, Health and Energy Conservation. Harvard University, 1981.

19 • Harris, J.C., Rumack, B.H., Aldrich, F.D.: Toxicology of urea formaldehyde and polyurethane foam insulation. JAMA 245:243, 1981.

20 • Kerfoot, E.J., Mooney, T.F.: Formaldehyde and paraformaldehyde study in funeral homes. Am. Industr. Hyg. Assoc. J.36:533-537, 1975.

21 • Kotin, P., Falk, H.L.: Atmospheric pollutants. Ann. Rev. Med. 15:233-254, 1964.

22 • Kreiss, K., Hodgson, M.J.: "Building-associated epidemics," Indoor Air Quality, CRC Press, Inc., Boca Raton, FL, 1984.

23 • Mokler, B.V., Wong, B.A., Snow, M.: "Respirable Particulates Generated by Pressurized Consumer Products: I. Experiment Method and General Characteristics". American Industrial Hygiene Association Journal. 40:330-338, April 1979.

24 • Mokler, B.V., Wong, B.A., Snow, M.J.: "Respirable Particulates Generated by Pressurized Consumer Products: I. Experimental Method and General Characteristics". American Industrial Hygiene Association Journal. 40:330-338, April, 1979.

25 • Murphy, G.B., Jr.:   Fiberglass pneumonosis. Arch. Environ. Health. 3:704, 1961.

26 • National Academy of Sciences: "Report on Indoor Air Quality." Washington, D.C.

27 • Newhouse, M.T.:   UFFI dust. Non-specific irritant only? Chest 82:511, 1982.

28 • Paliard, F., Roche, L., Exbrayat, C., Sprunch, E.:   Chronic asthma due to formaldehyde. Arch Mal Prof 10:528-530, 1949.

29 • Rader, J.:   Irritant effects of formaldehyde in anatomy laboratories. Analytic and experimental investigations. Doctoral Dissertation. University of Wurzburg, 1974.

30 • Sacca, J.D.:   Possible hazard with use of fiberglass air filters. Annals of Allergy, 34:2, February, 1975.

31 • Sakula, A.:   Formalin asthma in hospital laboratory staff. Lancet 2:816, 1975.

32 • Schepers, et. al.:   The biological action of fiberglass plastic dust. AMA Arch Ind Health 18:34, 1967.

33 • Ulsmer, A.G., Beall, J.R., Toxicity of Volatile Organic Compounds Used Indoor. C.P.S.C., Health Effects, 1981.

34 • U.S. Department of Energy, Office of Environment Programs. Indoor Air Quality Guide for Designers, Builders, and Users of Energy Efficient Residences. November, 1981.

35 • Willeke, Klaus, Generation of Aerosols. Mokler, B.V., Damon, E.G. Henderson, T.D., James, R.K., "Consumer Product Aerosals: Generation Characterization and Exposure Problems". Chapter 18: 379-398. Ann Arbor Science Publishers, Inc., Ann Arbor, 1980.

36 • Wright, G.W.:   Airborne fibrous glass particles. Arch. Environ. Health 16:175, 1968.

ALLERGY TESTING:

Bibliography Courtesy of American Academy Allergy & Immunology

1 • Black, A.P.: "A New Diagnostic method in Allergic Disease." Pediatrics, 17:716-723, 1956.

2 • Bryan, W.T.K., Bryan, M.P.: "The Application of In Vitro Cytotoxic Reactions to Clinical Diagnosis of Food Allergy." Laryngoscope, 70:810-824, 1960.

3 • Bryan, W.T.K., Bryan, M.P.: "Cytotoxic Reactions in the Diagnosis of food Allergy," Laryngoscope, 79:1453-1472, 1969.

4 • Bryan, W.T.k., Bryan, M.P. "Clinical Examples of Resolution of Some Idiopathic and Other Chronic Diseases by Careful Allergic Management." Laryngoscope, 82: 1231-1238, 1972.

5 • Chambers, V.V., Hudson, B.H., Glaser, J.: "A Study of Reactions of Human Polymorphonuclear Leukocytes to Various Allergens.: Journal of Allergy, 29:93-102, 1958.

6 • Lieberman, P., Crawford, L., Bjelland, J., Connell, B., Rice, M.: "controlled Study of the Cytotoxic Food Test." JAMA, 231:728-730, 1975.

7 • Benson, T.E., Arkins, J.A.: "Cytotoxic Testing for Food Allergy: Evaluation of Reproducibility and Correlation." Journal of Allergy and Clinical Immunology, 58:471-476, 1976.

8 • Lehman, C.W.: "The Leukoxytic Food Allergy Test: A Study of its Reliability and Reproducibility. Effect of Diet and Sublingual Food Drops on this Test." Annals of Allergy, 45:150-158, 1980.

9 • Report from the NCHCT. "Summary of Assessments, 1981." JAMA, 246:1499, 1981.

10 • American Academy of Allergy, "Position Statements — Controversial Techniques." Journal of Allergy and Clinical Immunology, 67:333-334, 1981.

11 • Grieco, M.H.: "Controversial Practices in Allergy." JAMA, 247:3106-3111, 1982.

12 • Goldbert, T.M.: "A Review of Controversial Diagnostic and Therapeutic techniques Employed in Allergy." Journal of Allergy and Clinical Immunology, 56:170-190, 1975.

13 • Updegraff, T.R.: "Food Allergy and Cytotoxic Tests." Ear, Nose & Throat Journal, 56:7-16, 1977.

14 • Boyles, J.H., Jr.: "The Validity of Using the Cytotoxic Food Test in Clinical Allergy." Ear, Nose & Throat, Reprint: 1-6, 1977.

15 • Ulett, G.A., Perry, S.G.: "Cytotoxic Testing and Leucocyte Increase as an Index to Food Sensitivity," Annals of Allergy, 33:17-76, 1974.

16 • Ruokonen, J., Holopainen, E., Palva, T., Palva, A.: "Secretory Otitis Media and Allergy." Allergy, 36:59-68.

17 • Holopainen, E., Palva, T., Stenberg, P., Buckman, A., Lehti, H., Ruokonen, J.: "Cytotoxic Leucocyte Reaction." Acta Otolaryngol, 89:222-226, 1980.

18 • Ulett, G.A., Perry, S.G.: "Cytotoxic Testing and Leucocyte Increase as an Index to Food Sensitivity II. Coffee and Tobacco." Annals of allergy, 34:150-160, 1975.

Judy Lee Bachman, Ph.D.

Dr. Bachman is the former Clinical Director of the Allergy Physician's Assistant Program at the School of Medicine at the University of California, San Diego. It was through this program that a body of knowledge evolved out of hundreds of environmental studies. Two other publications, "Ensuring Clean Air," and "Allergy Environment Control," are excerpted from this book. They are used as handouts by physicians and health educators. All three publications were developed on the principle that the allergic person can feel well most of the time by achieving balance under an appropriate treatment program, maintaining a healthy lifestyle and developing a home and work environment that reduces, or eliminates, exposures to allergens and air pollutants. The guidebook has been designed for allergy sufferers to participate in their treatment program as a team member.

NOTES

NOTES